Virtual Clinical Excursions—General Hospital

for

Christensen and Kockrow:
Foundations of Nursing
4th Edition

Virtual Clinical Excursions—General Hospital

for

Christensen and Kockrow:

Foundations of Nursing
4th Edition

prepared by

Ruth Eckenstein, RN, BS, M.ED
Program Specialist
Oklahoma Department of Career
and Technology Education
Stillwater, Oklahoma

Virtual Clinical Excursions Author and Software Design

Jay Shiro Tashiro, PhD, RN
Director of Systems Design
Wolfsong Informatics
Tucson, Arizona

Ellen Sullins, PhD
Director of Research
Wolfsong Informatics
Tucson, Arizona

Gina Long, RN, DNSc
Assistant Professor, Department of Nursing
College of Health Professions
Northern Arizona University
Flagstaff, Arizona

Software Development

Michael Kelly
Developer and Programmer
Michael M. Kelly and Associates
Flagstaff, Arizona

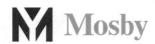

An Affiliate of Elsevier Science
St. Louis   London   Philadelphia   Sydney   Toronto

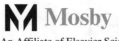

An Affiliate of Elsevier Science

11830 Westline Industrial Drive
St. Louis, Missouri 63146

Virtual Clinical Excursions for Christensen and Kockrow: ISBN 0-323-02472-6
Foundations of Nursing, 4th Edition
Copyright © 2003,   Mosby, Inc.   All rights reserved.

Notice

Pharmacology is an ever-changing field. Standard safety precautions must be followed, but as new research
and clinical experience broaden our knowledge, changes in treatment and drug therapy may become necessary or appropriate. Readers are advised to check the most current product information provided by the
manufacturer of each drug to be administered to verify the recommended dose, the method and duration of
administration, and contraindications. It is the responsibility of the licensed prescriber, relying on experience and knowledge of the patient, to determine dosages and the best treatment for each individual patient.
Neither the publisher nor the editor assumes any liability for any injury and/or damage to persons or prop-
erty arising from this publication.

The Publisher

First Edition 2003.

Executive Vice President, Nursing & Health Professions: Sally Schrefer
Editor, Nursing: Tom Wilhelm
Senior Developmental Editor: Jeff Downing
Editorial Assistant: Jennifer Anderson
Project Manager: Gayle May
Designer: Wordbench
Cover Art: Jyotika Schrof

Printed in the United States of America

Last digit is the print number: 9   8   7   6   5   4   3   2   1

Workbook
prepared by

Ruth Eckenstein, RN, BS, M.ED
Program Specialist
Oklahoma Department of Career
and Technology Education
Stillwater, Oklahoma

Textbook

Barbara Lauritsen Christensen, RN, MS
Nurse Educator
Mid-Plains Community College
North Platte, Nebraska

Elaine Oden Kockrow, RN, MS
Formerly, Nurse Educator
Mid-Plains Community College
North Platte, Nebraska

Contents

Getting Started

GETTING SET UP

■ MINIMUM SYSTEM REQUIREMENTS

Virtual Clinical Excursions—General Hospital is a hybrid CD, so it runs on both Macintosh and Windows platforms. To use *Virtual Clinical Excursions—General Hospital*, you will need one of the following systems:

- **Windows™**

    Windows XP, 2000, 98, 95, NT 4.0
    IBM-compatible computer
    Pentium II processor (or equivalent)
    300 MHz
    96 MB (minimum) of RAM
    800 × 600 screen size
    Thousands of colors
    100 MB hard drive space
    12× CD-ROM drive
    Soundblaster 16 soundcard compatibility
    Stereo speakers or headphones

- **Macintosh®**

    MAC OS 9.04
    Apple Power PC G3
    300 MHz
    96 MB (minimum) of RAM
    800 × 600 screen size
    Thousands of colors
    100 MB hard drive space
    12× CD-ROM drive
    Stereo speakers or headphones

Note: *Virtual Clinical Excursions—General Hospital* is not designed to function at a 256-color depth. You may need to go to the Control Panel and change the Display settings. Instructions on adjusting these settings may be found in the How to Adjust Your Monitor's Settings on p. 2 of this workbook.

■ INSTALLING *VIRTUAL CLINICAL EXCURSIONS—GENERAL HOSPITAL*

- **Windows™**

  1. Start Microsoft Windows and insert *Virtual Clinical Excursions—General Hospital* **Disk 1** in the CD-ROM drive.
  2. Click the **Start** button on the taskbar and select the **Run** option.
  3. Type d:\Windows 95 setup.exe or d:\Windows 98-XP setup.exe (depending on your operating system—where "d:\" is your CD-ROM drive) and press **OK**.
  4. Follow the on-screen instructions for installation.
  5. Remove *Virtual Clinical Excursions—General Hospital* **Disk 1** from your CD-ROM drive.
  6. Restart your computer.

- **Macintosh®**

  1. Insert *Virtual Clinical Excursions—General Hospital* **Disk 1** in the CD-ROM drive. The disk icon will appear on your desktop.
  2. Double-click on the disk icon.
  3. Double-click on the icon that reads **Install Virtual Clinical Excursions**.
  4. Follow the on-screen instructions for installation.
  5. Remove *Virtual Clinical Excursions—General Hospital* **Disk 1** from your CD-ROM drive.
  6. Restart your computer.

■ HOW TO ADJUST YOUR MONITOR'S SETTINGS (WINDOWS™ ONLY)

- **Windows 95/98/SE/ME/2000**

  1. Click the **Start** button and go to **Settings** on the pop-up menu. Click on **Control Panel**.
  2. When the Control Panel window opens, double-click on the **Display** icon.
  3. You will now be presented with the Display Properties window. Click on the **Settings** tab (on the right). Below the image of the monitor, you will see on the left the **Color** palette. (You should change this to **High Color [16 bit]** by selecting it from the drop-down menu. You will need to restart your computer to do this.) On the right is the desktop area. Left-click and hold down on the slider button and move it to 800 by 600 pixels. Now click **OK**.
  4. Windows will ask you to confirm the change; click **OK**. Your screen will resize and Windows will again ask you whether you want to keep these new settings. Click **Yes**.

- **Windows XP**

  1. Click the **Start** button; then click **Control Panel** on the pop-up menu.
  2. Click **Display**. If Display does not appear, click **Switch to Classic View**; then click on **Display** icon.
  3. From the Display Properties dialog box, select the **Settings** tab.
  4. Under Screen Resolution, click and drag the sliding bar to adjust the desktop size to 800 x 600 pixels.
  5. Under Color Quality, choose **High** or **Highest**.
  6. Click **Apply**. If you approve of the new settings, click **Yes**.

■ HOW TO ACCESS PATIENTS

Unlike previous VCE products that presented all of the patients on one disk, *Virtual Clinical Excursions—General Hospital* includes patients on both disks. Both of the patients on the Pediatric Floor (Floor 3) are found on Disk 1, which you used to install the program. The remaining patients—including three patients in the Medical-Surgical-Telemetry Unit (Floor 6), one patient in the Intensive Care Unit (Floor 5), and one patient who spends time in the Medical-Surgical-Telemetry Unit (Floor 6) and in the Surgery Department (Floor 4)—are located on Disk 2. When you want to work with any of the seven patients in the virtual hospital, follow these steps:

- **Windows™**

  1. Insert the *Virtual Clinical Excursions—General Hospital* disk that contains the patient you want to work with into your CD-ROM drive.
  2. Double-click on the icon **Shortcut to Virtual Clinical Excursions**, which can be found on your desktop. This will load and run the program.

- **Macintosh®**

  1. Insert the *Virtual Clinical Excursions—General Hospital* disk that contains the patient you want to work with into your CD-ROM drive.
  2. Double-click on the icon **Shortcut to Virtual Clinical Excursions**, which can be found on your desktop. This will load and run the program.

■ QUALITY OF VISUALS, SPEED, AND COMMON PROBLEMS

Virtual Clinical Excursions—General Hospital uses the Apple QuickTime media layer system. This includes QuickTime Video and QuickTime VR Video, which allow for high-quality graphics and digital video. The graphics seen in the *Virtual Clinical Excursions—Medical-Surgical* courseware should be of high quality with rich color. If the movies and graphics appear blocky or grainy, check to see whether your video card is set to "thousands of colors."

Note: Virtual Clinical Excursions—General Hospital is not designed to function at a 256-color depth. To adjust your monitor's settings, see instructions on p. 2.

The system should respond quickly and smoothly. In particular, you should not see any jerky motions or experience unusual delays as you move through the virtual hospital settings, interact with patients, or access information resources. If you notice slow, jerky, or delayed software responses, it may mean that your particular system requires additional RAM, your processor does not meet the basic requirements, or your hard drive is full or too fragmented. If the videos appear banded or subject to "breakup," you may need to find an updated video driver for the computer's video card. Please consult the manufacturer of the video card or computer for additional video drivers for your machine.

If you are experiencing misplacement of text or cursors in the Electronic Patient Record (EPR), it is likely that your computer operating system has enabled font smoothing. Please turn font smoothing off by following these instructions:

- **Windows™**

  From the Control Panel window click on **Display** and then select the **Appearance** tab. Click on **Effects** and make sure the box next to "Smooth Edges of Screen Fonts" option is unselected.

- **Macintosh®**

  From the desktop, click on the **Apple** icon in the upper left corner. From the drop-down menu, select **Control Panel**; then select **Appearance**. Click on the **Fonts** tab and make sure the selection box next to "Smooth all fonts on screen" is unselected.

Virtual Clinical Excursions—General Hospital uses Adobe Acrobat Reader version 5 to display information in certain places in the simulation. If you cannot see any information when accessing the Charts, Medication Administration Record (MAR), or Kardex, it is likely that Adobe Acrobat Reader was not installed properly when you installed *Virtual Clinical Excursions—General Hospital*. To remedy this, you can manually install Acrobat Reader from the *Virtual Clinical Excursions—General Hospital* **Disk 1**. Double-click the **Adobe Acrobat Reader** installer (ar505enu.exe) on the disk and follow the on-screen instructions. Once the installer has finished installing Acrobat Reader, restart your computer and then resume your use of *Virtual Clinical Excursions—General Hospital*.

■ TECHNICAL SUPPORT

Technical support for this product is available at no charge by calling the Technical Support Hotline between 9 a.m. and 5 p.m. (Central Time), Monday through Friday. Inside the United States, call 1-800-692-9010. Outside the United States, call 314-872-8370.

Trademarks: Windows™ is a registered trademark.

A QUICK TOUR

Welcome to *Virtual Clinical Excursions—General Hospital*, a virtual hospital setting in which you can work with seven patient simulations and also learn to access and evaluate the health information resources that are essential for high-quality patient care.

The virtual hospital, **Canyon View Regional Medical Center**, is a multistory teaching hospital with a Well-Child Clinic, Pediatric Floor, Surgery Department, Intensive Care Unit, and a Medical-Surgical Floor with a Telemetry Unit. You will have access to the adult patients in the Intensive Care Unit and on the Medical-Surgical Floor. One patient will also spend time in the Surgery Department, where you can follow her through a perioperative experience.

Although each floor plan in the medical center is different, each is based on a realistic hospital architecture modeled from a composite of several hospital settings. All floors have:

- A Nurses' Station
- Patients, seen either in examination areas or in their inpatient rooms
- Patient records, including a Chart, Kardex plan of care, Medication Administration Record, and Electronic Patient Record accessed through a simulated computerized system.

■ BEFORE YOU START

When you use *Virtual Clinical Excursions—General Hospital*, make sure you have your textbook nearby to consult topic areas as needed. Also make sure that you have both disks to run the simulations. If you have not already installed your *VCE—General Hospital* software, do so now by following the steps outlined in **Getting Set Up** at the beginning of this workbook.

■ ENTERING THE HOSPITAL AND SELECTING A CLINICAL ROTATION

To begin your tour of Canyon View Regional Medical Center, insert your *Virtual Clinical Excursions—General Hospital* Disk 2 and double-click on the desktop icon **Shortcut to VCE—General Hospital**. Wait for the hospital entrance screen to appear (see below). This is your signal that the program is ready to run. Your first task is to get to the unit where you will be caring for patients and to let someone know when you arrive at the unit. As in any multistory hospital, you will enter the hospital lobby area, take an elevator to your assigned unit, and sign in at the Nurses' Station.

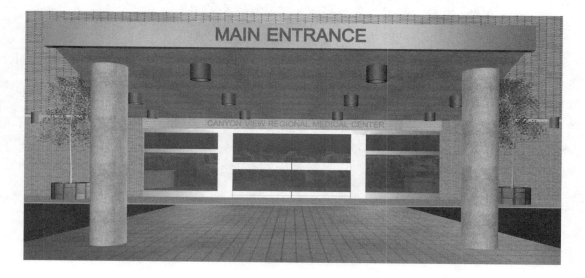

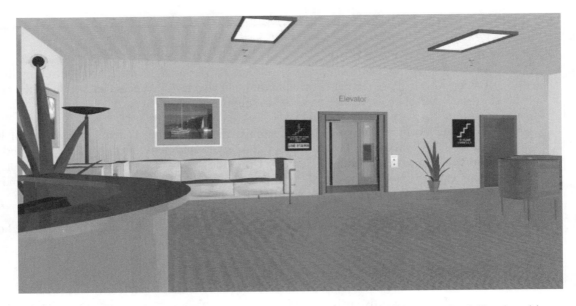

Let's practice getting to your unit in Canyon View Regional Medical Center by following this sequence:

- Click on the hospital entrance door and you will find yourself in the hospital lobby on the first floor (see above).
- Across the lobby, you will see an elevator with a blinking red light. Click on the open doorway and you will be transported into the elevator (see below).
- Now click on the panel on the right side of the doorway. The panel will expand to reveal buttons that allow you to go to the other floors of the hospital (see p. 7).
- Slowly run your cursor across the buttons to familiarize yourself with the different floors and units of the hospital.

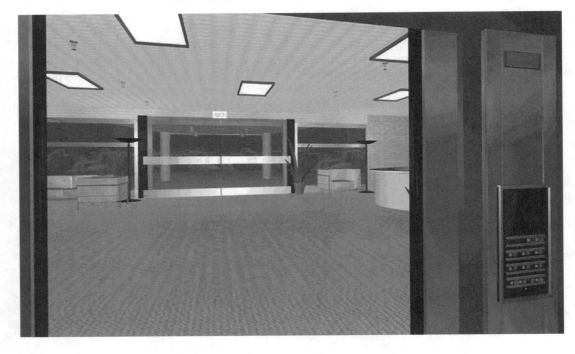

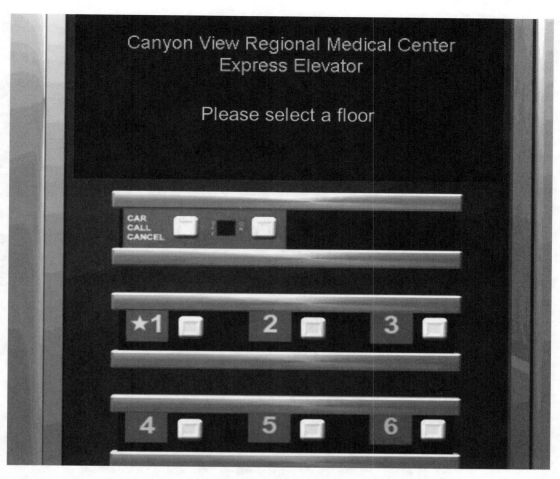

Since you are in a medical-surgical rotation, you will not be able to visit the Well-Child Clinic. However, you can work with two patients on the Pediatric Floor (Disk 1), one patient in the Intensive Care Unit (Disk 2), three patients on the Medical-Surgical/Telemetry Floor (Disk 2), and one who spends time on both the Medical-Surgical/Telemetry Floor and in the Surgery Department (Disk 2).

Now, go to a unit and sign in for patient care. With Disk 2 in your CD-ROM drive, try this:

- Click on the button for the Medical-Surgical/Telemetry Floor, which is Floor 6.
- The elevator takes you to that floor and opens onto a virtual unit with a Nurses' Station in the center and rooms arrayed around the Nurses' Station.
- Click on the **Nurses' Station** and you will be transported behind its counter.
- If you click and hold the mouse button down, you can get a 360° view of the Medical-Surgical/Telemetry floor by dragging your mouse left or right. With the button still held down, drag to the left, then up, then down. You get a complete view of the Nurses' Station and the floor (see p. 8).
- Take a few minutes to familiarize yourself with the Nurses' Station. Find the two computers, one of which has **Login** on its screen. This is the computer that allows you to select a patient. The other computer is the **Electronic Patient Records** terminal. As you look around the Nurses' Station, you also will see the patient Charts, the Kardex plan of care notebooks, and the Medication Administration Record notebook (labeled MAR).

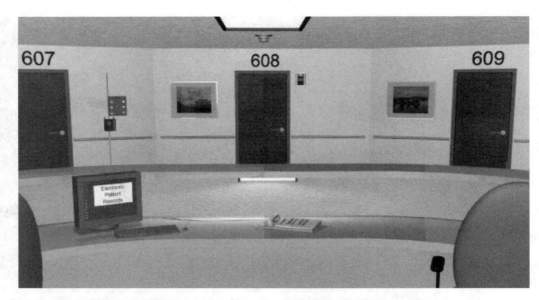

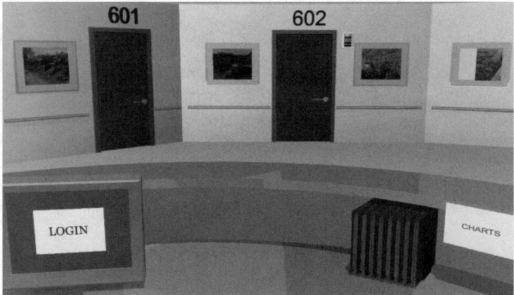

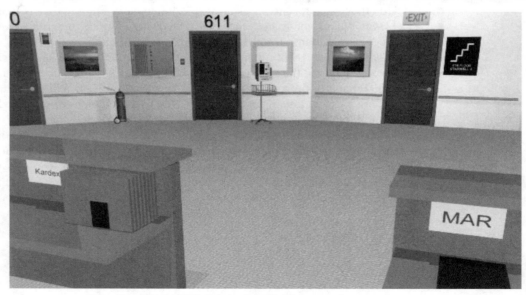

■ WORKING WITH PATIENTS

In *Virtual Clinical Excursions—General Hospital*, the Medical-Surgical/Telemetry floor can be visited between 07:00 and 15:00, but a user can see only one patient at a time and then only in blocks of time. We call these blocks "periods of care." In any of the Medical-Surgical/Telemetry floor scenarios, you can select a patient and a period of care by accessing the Supervisor's (Login) Computer. Double-click on this computer to open the sign-in screen, which contains a box with instructions. Click the **Login** button and you will see a screen that lists the patients on this floor and the periods of care in which you can visit and work with them. Again, only one patient can be selected at a time. When work is completed on that patient, you can select another period of care for that patient or another patient.

Note: During a patient simulation you may receive an on-screen message informing you that the current period of care has ended. If this occurs and you have not yet completed the assigned activities (or if you want to review part of the simulation), you can return to the Supervisor's Computer and sign in again for the same patient and period of care. When the Warning screen appears, click **Erase**. On the other hand, if you simply want to review the data you entered during that period of care, you can sign in for the same patient in a later time period and review data in the EPR. Please note that this option doesn't apply to the final period of care. If you are working with a patient during the last period of care, make sure you keep an eye on the on-screen clock and are aware of how much time is remaining.

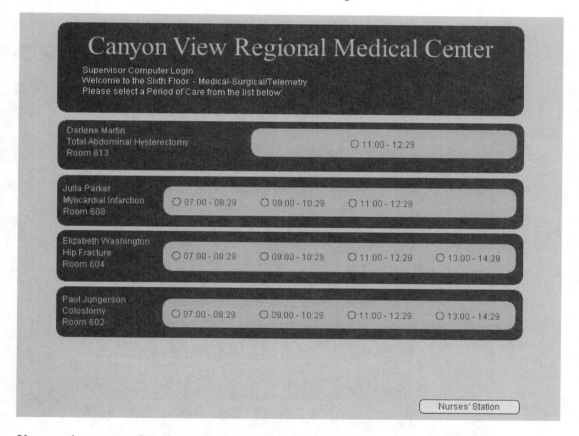

You can choose any of the four patients on this floor (but only one at a time). For each patient you will select a period of care. Three of the patients (Julia Parker, Elizabeth Washington, and Paul Jungerson) can be seen during four periods of care: 07:00–08:29, 09:00–10:29, 11:00–12:29, and 13:00–14:29. You will follow the fourth patient, Darlene Martin, through a Perioperative Rotation. You see her first in the Surgery Department (Floor 4) for a Preoperative Interview (conducted two days prior to surgery). She then goes to the Surgery Department for preoperative care, surgery, and a period in the PACU (09:30–10:29). After leaving PACU, she is transferred to the Medical-Surgical/Telemetry Floor (Floor 6) at 11:00, and you can see her on that floor from 11:00–12:29. There is one patient, James Story, in the Intensive Care Unit (Floor 6).

There are two patients (De Olp and Maria Ortiz) on the Pediatric Floor. Although the patients in the Surgery Department (Floor 4), Intensive Care Unit (Floor 5), and the Medical-Surgical/ Telemetry Floor (Floor 6) are all found on Disk 2, the patients on the Pediatric Floor are found on Disk 1. Here are the steps to follow when you need to swap disks:

- If you are currently signed in for a patient, go to the Supervisor's (Login) Computer and sign out. Return to the Nurses' Station.
- Leave the Nurses' Station and enter the elevator. Once you are inside the elevator, remove the disk from your CD-ROM drive and replace it with the other disk.
- Click on the button of the floor number where you need to go.

If you attempt to access the Pediatric Floor (Floor 3) while Disk 2 is in your CD-ROM drive, the computer will eject the disk and prompt you to insert Disk 1 to continue (see below). Likewise, if you attempt to access the Surgery Department, ICU, or the Medical-Surgical/Telemetry Floor while Disk 1 is in your CD-ROM drive, the disk will be ejected and the computer will prompt you to insert Disk 2 to continue.

(*Note:* The process of selecting patients is basically the same on all floors of Canyon View Regional Medical Center, although the available periods of care in the Surgery Department are different from those on the other floors. You will observe this when you visit the other floors.)

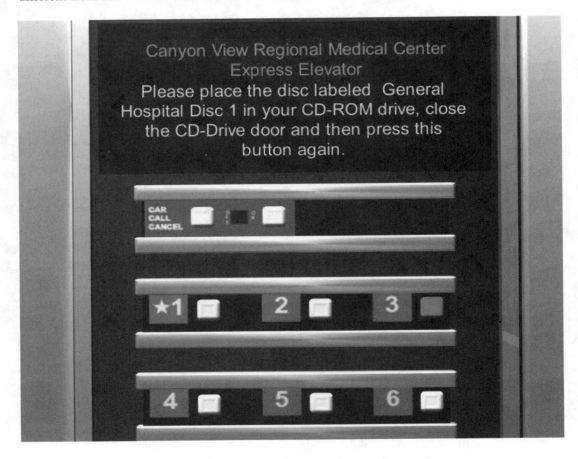

■ **PATIENT LIST**

◆ **Floor 3: Pediatric Floor (Disk 1)**

- Maria Ortiz (Room 308)
  Maria is an 8-year-old child who was admitted from the Emergency Department with an acute exacerbation of asthma. She has a 2-year history of asthma. Past acute exacerbation have been treated with Prelone.

- De Olp (Room 310)
  De is a 6-year-old girl who entered the hospital 4 days ago. A bone marrow aspiration confirmed a diagnosis of acute lymphoblastic leukemia. She has had a lumbar puncture for assessment of cerebral spinal fluid, intrathecal chemotherapy, and placement of a Port-a-Cath for administering additional chemotherapy agents.

◆ **Floor 4: Surgery Department (Disk 2)**

- Darlene Martin
  Ms. Martin is a 49-year-old female who begins Tuesday in the Surgery Department to prepare for a total abdominal hysterectomy. She has been suffering from irregular periods and an enlarged uterus over the past six months, which has caused endometrial hyperplasia. A few days before her surgery, she had a preoperative interview. On Tuesday morning she enters a period of preoperative care, then undergoes a hysterectomy. After a period in the Post-Anesthesia Care Unit (PACU), she is transferred to the Medical-Surgical/Telemetry Floor.

◆ **Floor 5: Intensive Care Unit (Disk 2)**

- James Story (Room 512)
  Mr. Story is a 42-year-old male who arrived in the Emergency Department complaining of shortness of breath, increasing weakness with a tingling sensation in his extremities, nausea, recent onset of diarrhea, lower leg edema, and a significantly edematous right arm. Mr. Story has type 1 (insulin-dependent) diabetes mellitus and has been undergoing hemodialysis treatment for almost a year. During his stay, he begins experiencing renal failure.

◆ **Floor 6: Medical-Surgical/Telemetry Floor (Disk 2)**

- Paul Jungerson (Room 602)
  Mr. Jungerson is a 61-year-old male who is recovering from a colon resection. He has a history of diverticulitis, hypertension, pneumonia, and chronic ankle pain.

- Elizabeth Washington (Room 604)
  Ms. Washington is a 63-year-old female who was admitted following an auto accident in which she fractured her hip. She has a history of hypertension and asthma.

- Julia Parker (Room 608)
  Ms. Parker is a 51-year-old female who presented to the Emergency Department with indigestion and mid-back pain. She has a history of hypertension, type 2 diabetes, hyperlipidemia, and obesity. During her stay, she undergoes a heart catheterization and angioplasty, before suffering a myocardial infarction.

- Darlene Martin (Room 613)
  Remember Darlene Martin, the surgical patient? (See Floor 4 above.) After a period in the PACU, Ms. Martin is transferred to the Medical-Surgical/Telemetry Floor.

■ VISITING A PATIENT

Each time you sign in for a new patient and period of care, you enter the simulation at the start of that period of care. The simulations are constructed so that you can conduct a fairly complete assessment of your patient in the first 30 minutes of each period of care. However, after completing a general survey, you should begin to focus your assessments on specific areas. For example, within one period of care you should not do a head-to-toe examination each time you come into a patient's room. Instead, conduct a complete physical at the start of a period of care, then select assessments that are appropriate for your patient's current condition and are based on how that condition is changing. Just as in the real world, a patient's data will change over time as the patient improves or deteriorates. Even if a patient remains stable, there will be diurnal variations in physiology, and these will be reflected in changes in assessment data.

As soon as you sign in to begin working with a patient, a clock appears on screen to help you keep track of time. The clock, which operates in "real time," is located in the bottom left-hand corner of the screen when you are in the Nurses' Station and in the top right-hand corner when you are in the patient's room.

To become familiar with some of the learning resources in *Virtual Clinical Excursions—General Hospital*, insert Disk 2 in your CD-ROM drive, go to Floor 6, select Elizabeth Washington, and choose the 07:00–08:29 period of care. Then click on the button in the lower right corner labeled **Nurses' Station**. This procedure will select the patient and time period for your work. You are then automatically sent to a Case Overview, which provides a short video in which your preceptor introduces the patient. There is also a button labeled **Assignment**. Clicking on this button will open a summary sheet that provides information about the patient and guidance for your work in the simulation.

After completing the Case Overview, you can enter the simulation by clicking on the **Nurses' Station** button in the lower right corner of the screen. This will take you back to the Nurses' Station, where you can begin working with your patient. Remember three things:

- You must select a patient and period of care before any of that patient's simulation and data become available to you.
- Just as in the real world, the Nurses' Station is the base from which you can access patient records and from which you go onto the floor to visit a patient.
- Before you can access another patient simulation, you must go back to the Supervisor's (Login) Computer and follow the procedure to sign out from your current period of care.

Now that you have signed in to care for a patient, Elizabeth Washington, you have several choices. You can enter Elizabeth's room and work with your preceptor to assess the patient. You can review her patient records, which include her Chart, a Kardex plan of care, her active Medication Administration Record (MAR), or the Electronic Patient Record (EPR), all of which contain data that have been collected since Elizabeth entered the hospital. You may know that some hospitals have only paper records and others have only electronic records. Canyon View Regional Medical Center, the virtual hospital, has a combination of paper records (the patient's Chart, Kardex, and MAR) and electronic records (the EPR).

Let's begin by becoming more familiar with the Nurses' Station screen. In the upper left-hand corner, find a menu with these five buttons:

- Patient Care
- Planning Care
- Patient Records
- Case Conference
- Clinical Review

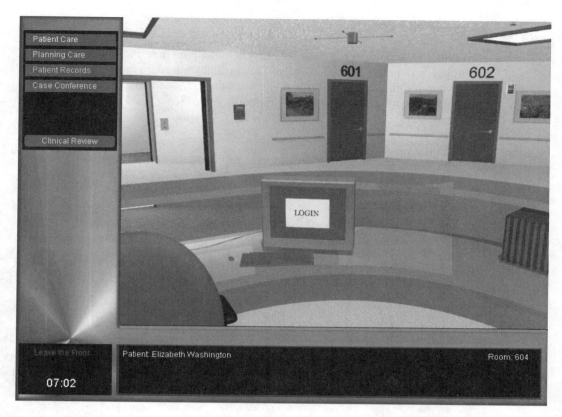

One at a time, single-click on these buttons to reveal drop-down menus with additional options for each item. First, click on **Patient Care**. Two options are available for this item: **Case Overview** and **Data Collection**. You completed the Case Overview after signing in for Ms. Washington, but you can always go back to review it. For example, you might want to return there and click the **Assignment** button to review the summary of Ms. Washington's care up to the start of your shift—or to remind yourself what tasks you have been asked to complete.

◆ **Data Collection**

To conduct an assessment of your patient, click **Patient Care** and then **Data Collection** from the drop-down menu. This will take you into a small anteroom (part of the patient's room) with a sink, laundry bin, and biohazards waste receptacle. *Note:* You can also enter this anteroom by clicking on the outer door of Ms. Washington's room (Room 604). To visit your patient, complete these steps:

- First *wash your hands!* Click on the sink once to indicate you are beginning to wash. Click again to indicate you are finished washing.
- Now click on the curtain to the right of the sink and enter the patient's room.

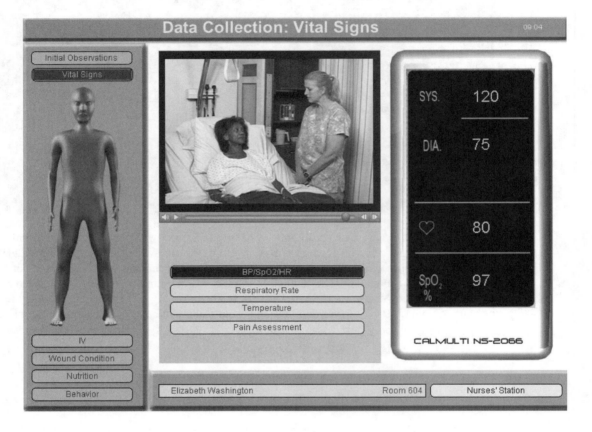

Once in the patient's room, your screen is equipped with various tools you can use for data collection. In the center of the screen, you will see a still frame of your patient. Along the left side of the screen are buttons and a body model that allow you to access learning activities in which your preceptor conducts different types of assessments. Try clicking on the buttons and different body parts. (Note that the body model rotates once your cursor touches it. As you move your cursor over the model, various body parts are highlighted in orange.)

What happened when you clicked on the buttons or body parts? Many of the buttons open options for additional assessments—these always appear below the video screen. Likewise, clicking on a highlighted area of the body model opens options for additional assessments. The body model serves two purposes. First, it provides a way for you to develop a sense of what assessments and physiologic systems are associated with different areas of the human body. Second, it acts as a quick navigational tool that allows you to focus on certain types of assessments.

Note that the body model is a "generic" figure without specific sexual or racial characteristics. However, we encourage you to always think about your patients as unique individuals. The body model is simply a tool designed to help you develop assessment skills by body area and navigate quickly though the simulation's learning activities. Review the diagram below to become familiar with the available Data Collection buttons and the additional options that appear when you click each button and body area.

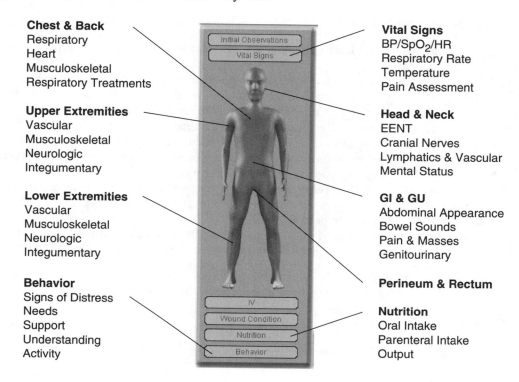

Chest & Back
Respiratory
Heart
Musculoskeletal
Respiratory Treatments

Upper Extremities
Vascular
Musculoskeletal
Neurologic
Integumentary

Lower Extremities
Vascular
Musculoskeletal
Neurologic
Integumentary

Behavior
Signs of Distress
Needs
Support
Understanding
Activity

Vital Signs
BP/SpO$_2$/HR
Respiratory Rate
Temperature
Pain Assessment

Head & Neck
EENT
Cranial Nerves
Lymphatics & Vascular
Mental Status

GI & GU
Abdominal Appearance
Bowel Sounds
Pain & Masses
Genitourinary

Perineum & Rectum

Nutrition
Oral Intake
Parenteral Intake
Output

Whenever you click on an assessment button, either a video or still photo will be activated in the center of the screen. For some activities, data obtained during assessment are shown in a box to the right of that frame (see p. 14). For other assessment options, you must collect data yourself by observing the video—in these cases, no data appear in the box. You can always replay a video by simply reclicking the assessment button of the activity you wish to see again.

The *Virtual Clinical Excursions—General Hospital* patient simulations were constructed by expert nurses to be as realistic as possible. As previously mentioned, the data for every patient will change through time. During the first 30 minutes of a period of care, you will generally find that all assessment options will give you data on the patient. However, after that period, some assessments may no longer be a high priority for a patient. The expert nurses who created the patient simulations let you know when an assessment area is not a high priority by sending you a short message. These messages appear in the box on the right side of the screen, where data are normally listed. Some examples of messages you might receive include "Please rethink your priorities for assessment of this patient" and "Your assessment should be focused on other areas at this time."

To leave the patient's room, click on the **Nurses' Station** button in the bottom right-hand corner of the screen. Note that this takes you back through the anteroom, where you must wash your hands before leaving. Once you have washed your hands, click on the outer door to return to the Nurses' Station.

Now, let's review what you just learned and try a few quick exercises to get a sense of how the Data Collection learning activities become available to you. You are already signed in to care for Elizabeth Washington, who was admitted following an auto accident in which her hip was fractured. Reenter her room from the Nurses' Station by clicking on **Patient Care** and then on **Data Collection**. You are now in the sink area of the patient's room, so wash your hands and click on the curtain to see the patient.

Start your patient care by collecting Ms. Washington's vital signs.

- Click on **Vital Signs**. Four assessment options will appear below the picture of the patient.
- Click on **BP/SpO₂/HR**. Watch the video as your preceptor measures blood pressure, oxygen saturation, and heart rate on a noninvasive multipurpose monitor. Record Ms. Washington's data for these attributes in the chart below.
- Now click on **Respiratory Rate**. This time, after a video plays, a "breathing" body model appears on the right. Measure Ms. Washington's respiratory rate by counting the respirations of the body model for the period of time your instructor recommends. Record your estimate of her respiratory rate below.
- Next, click on **Temperature**. First, you will see your preceptor measuring Ms. Washington's temperature; then the thermometer reading appears in the frame to the right. Record her temperature.
- Finally, assess Ms. Washington's pain by clicking on **Pain Assessment**. Note your interpretation of her pain. If she is in pain, record her pain level and characteristics.

Vital Signs	Time
Blood pressure	
SpO₂	
Heart rate	
Respiratory rate	
Temperature	
Pain rating	

Once you have collected Ms. Washington's vital signs, begin a lower extremities examination. Point your cursor to the leg area of the body model. Click anywhere on the orange highlighted area. Four new options now appear below the picture of your patient.

- Click on **Vascular**. Observe the video and review the data you obtain from this examination.
- Now click on **Neurologic**. Is Ms. Washington experiencing any numbness or tingling in her arms or legs?

You have now collected vital signs data and conducted a limited lower extremities assessment of Ms. Washington. As previously mentioned, most of the assessments combine a video or still photo of the patient with data that are collected for the respective assessment. Other assessments simply provide a video, and you must collect data from the nurse-patient interaction. For example, many of the pain assessments consist of the nurse asking the patient to rate his or her pain and the patient responding with a rating. Some of the behavior assessments also require that you listen to the nurse-patient interaction and make a decision about the patient's condition, needs, or psychosocial attributes.

When you visit patients in the Surgery Department, you will notice slightly different assessment options for some periods of care. However, the same types of interactions are always available. When you click on a button or area of the body model, you will be able to access a variety of patient assessments. If a video is shown, it can always be replayed by clicking on the assessment button.

■ HOW TO FIND AND ACCESS A PATIENT'S RECORDS

So far, you have visited a patient and practiced collecting data. Now you will examine the types of available patient records and learn how to access them. The records include the patient Charts, Medication Administration Record (MAR), Kardex plan of care, and Electronic Patient Record (EPR).

You are still signed in for Elizabeth Washington on the Medical-Surgical/Telemetry Floor, so let's explore her records. From the Nurses' Station, each type of patient record can be accessed in two ways. Practice both methods and choose the pathway you prefer. The first option is to use the menu in the upper left corner of the screen. First, click on **Patient Records**; this reveals a drop-down menu. Then select the type of patient record you wish to review by clicking on one of these options:

- **EPR**—Electronic Patient Record
- **Chart**—The patient's chart
- **Kardex**—A Kardex plan of care
- **MAR**—The current Medication Administration Record

You can also access patient records by clicking on various objects in the Nurses' Station. On the counter inside the station you will find a set of charts, a set of Kardex plans of care, a Medication Administration Record notebook, and a computer that houses the Electronic Patient Record system. All objects inside the Nurses' Station are labeled for quick recognition.

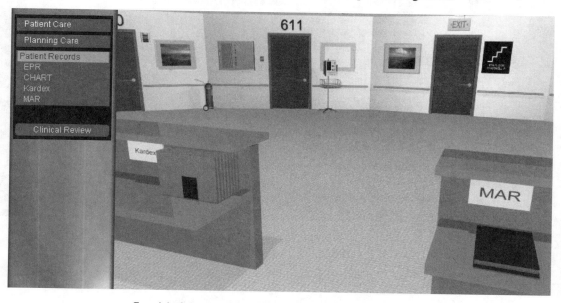

Chart

To open Ms. Washington's chart, click on **Chart** in the **Patient Records** drop-down menu—or click on the stack of Charts inside the Nurses' Station. Colored tabs at the bottom of the screen allow you to navigate through the following sections of the chart:

- History & Physical
- Nursing History
- Admissions Records
- Physician Orders
- Progress Notes
- Laboratory Reports
- X-Rays & Diagnostics
- Operative Reports
- Medication Records
- Consults
- Rehabilitation & Therapy
- Social Services
- Miscellaneous

To flip forward in the chart, select any available tab. Once you have moved beyond the first tab (History & Physical), a **Flip Back** icon appears just above the red cross in the lower right corner. Click on **Flip Back** to return to earlier sections of the chart. The data for each patient's chart are updated during a shift; updates occur at the start of a period of care. Note that some of the records in the chart are several pages long. You will need to scroll down to read all of the pages in some sections of the chart.

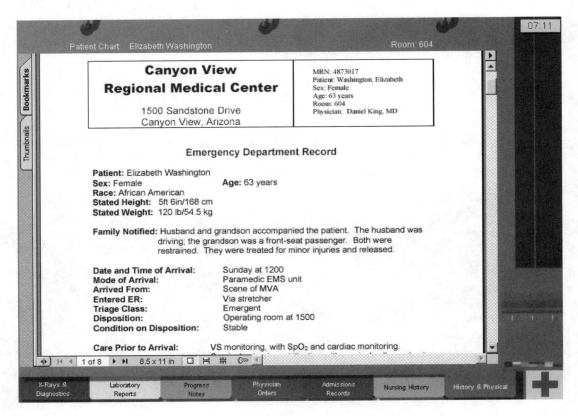

Flipping forward and back through the various sections is accomplished by clicking on the tabs or on the **Flip Back** icon. To close a patient's chart, click on the **Nurses' Station** icon in the lower right corner of the screen.

Medication Administration Record (MAR)

The notebook under the MAR sign in the Nurses' Station contains the active Medication Administration Record for each patient. This record lists the current 24-hour medication orders for each patient. Double-click on the MAR to open it like a notebook. (*Remember:* You can also access the MAR through the Patient Records menu.) Once open, the MAR has tabs that allow you to select patients by room number. Each MAR lists the following information for every medication a patient is receiving:

- Medication name
- Route and dosage of medication
- Time to administer medication

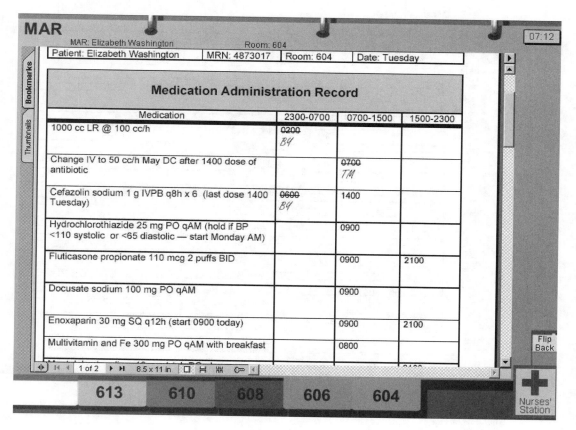

MAR: Elizabeth Washington Room: 604

Patient: Elizabeth Washington	MRN: 4873017	Room: 604	Date: Tuesday

Medication Administration Record

Medication	2300-0700	0700-1500	1500-2300
1000 cc LR @ 100 cc/h	0200 BY		
Change IV to 50 cc/h May DC after 1400 dose of antibiotic		0700 TM	
Cefazolin sodium 1 g IVPB q8h x 6 (last dose 1400 Tuesday)	0600 BY	1400	
Hydrochlorothiazide 25 mg PO qAM (hold if BP <110 systolic or <65 diastolic — start Monday AM)		0900	
Fluticasone propionate 110 mcg 2 puffs BID		0900	2100
Docusate sodium 100 mg PO qAM		0900	
Enoxaparin 30 mg SQ q12h (start 0900 today)		0900	2100
Multivitamin and Fe 300 mg PO qAM with breakfast		0800	

1 of 2   8.5 x 11 in

613   610   608   606   604

Scroll down to be sure you have read all the data. As with the patient charts, flip forward and back through the MAR by clicking on the patient room tabs or on the **Flip Back** icon. *Note:* Unlike the patient's Chart, which allows you to access data *only* for the patient for whom you are signed in, the MAR allows access to the data for *all* patients on the floor. Because the MAR is arranged numerically by patient room number, it is important that you remember to click on the correct tab for your current patient rather than reading the first record that appears on opening the MAR.

The MAR is updated at the start of every period of care. To close the MAR, click on the **Nurses' Station** icon in the lower right corner of the screen.

Kardex Plan of Care

Most hospitals keep a notebook in the Nurses' Station with each patient's plan of care. Canyon View Regional Medical Center's simplified plan of care is a three-page document modeled after the Kardex forms often used in hospitals. Access the Kardex through the drop-down menu (click **Patient Records**, then **Kardex**), or click on the folders beneath the Kardex sign in the Nurses' Station. *Note:* Like the MAR, the Kardex allows access to the plans of care for *all* patients on the floor. Side tabs allow you to select the patient's care plan by room number. Remember to click on the tab for your current patient rather than reading the first plan of care that appears after opening the Kardex. Scroll down to read all of the pages.

A Flip Back icon appears in the upper right corner once you have moved past the first patient's Kardex. Use the Nurses' Station icon in the bottom right corner to return to close the Kardex.

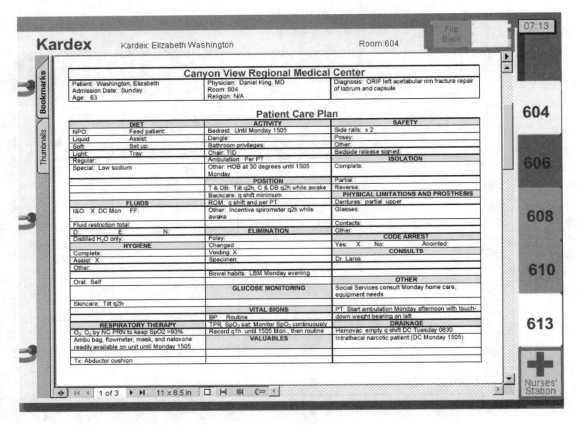

Electronic Patient Record (EPR)

Some patient records are kept in a computerized system called the Electronic Patient Record (EPR). Although some hospitals have only limited electronic patient records—or none at all—most hospitals are moving toward computerized or electronic patient record systems.

The Canyon View EPR was designed to represent a composite of commercial versions used in existing hospitals and clinics. If you have already used an EPR in a hospital, you will recognize the basic features of all commercial or custom-designed EPRs. If you have not used an EPR, the Canyon View system will give you an introduction to a basic computerized record system.

You can use the EPR to review data already recorded for a patient—or to enter assessment data that you have collected. The EPR is continually updated. For example, when you begin working with a patient for the 11:00–12:29 period of care, you have access to all the data for that patient up to 11:00. The EPR contains all data collected on the patient from the moment he or she entered the hospital. The Canyon View EPR allows you to examine how data for different attributes have changed during the time the patient has been in the hospital. You may also examine data for all of a patient's attributes at a particular time. Remember, the Canyon View EPR is fully functional, as in a real hospital. Just as in real life, you can enter data during the period of care in which you are working, but you cannot change data from a previous period of care.

You can access the EPR once you have signed in for a patient. Use the Patient Records menu or find the computer in the Nurses' Station with **Electronic Patient Records** on the screen. To access a patient's EPR:

- Select the EPR option on the drop-down menu (click **Patient Records**, then **EPR**) or double-click on the EPR computer screen. This will open the access screen.
- Type in the password—this will always be **nurse2b**—but *Do Not Hit Return* after entering the password.
- Click on the **Access Records** button.
- If you make a mistake, simply delete the password, reenter it, and click **Access Records**.

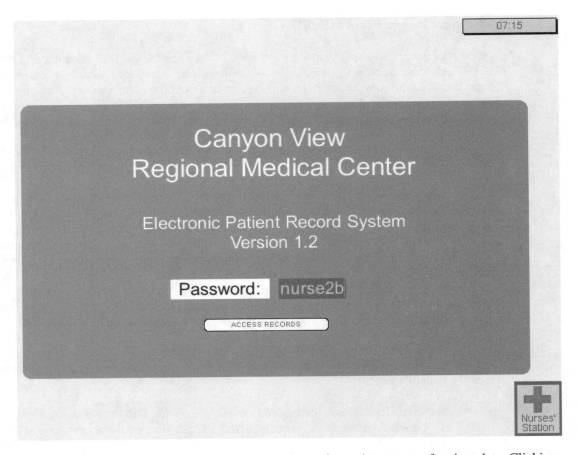

At the bottom of the EPR screen, you will see buttons for various types of patient data. Clicking on a button will bring up a field of attributes and the data for those attributes. You may notice that the data for some attributes appear as codes. The appropriate codes (and interpretations) for any attributes can be found in the code box on the far right side of the screen. Remember that every hospital or clinic selects its own codes. The codes used by Canyon View Regional Medical Center may be different from ones you have used or seen in clinical rotations. However, you will have to adjust to the various codes used by the clinical settings in which you work, so *Virtual Clinical Excursions—General Hospital* gives you some practice using a system different from one you may already know. The different data fields available in the EPR are:

- Vital Signs
- Neurologic
- Musculoskeletal
- Respiratory
- Cardiovascular
- GI & GU
- IV
- Equipment
- Drains & Tubes
- Wounds & Dressings
- Hygiene
- Safety & Comfort
- Behavior & Activity
- Intake & Output

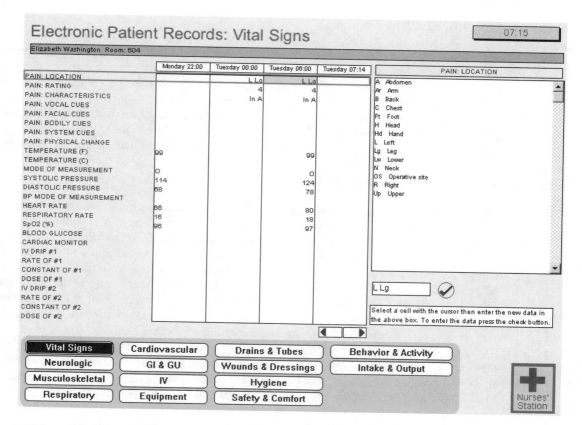

Click on **Vital Signs** and review the vital signs data for Elizabeth Washington. If you want to enter data you have collected for a particular attribute (such as pain characteristics), click on the data field in which the attribute is found. (Pain characteristics are found in the Vital Signs field.) Then click on the specific attribute line, and move the highlighted box to the current time cell. Blue arrows in the lower right corner move you left and right within the EPR data fields. Once the highlighted box is in the correct time cell, type in the code for your patient's pain characteristics in the box at the lower right side of the screen, just to the left of the check mark (√). Be sure to use the codes listed in the code box in the data entry area. Once you have typed the data in this box, click on the check mark (√) to enter and save them in the patient's record. The data will appear in the time cell for the attribute you have selected.

When you are ready to leave the EPR, click on the **Nurses' Station** icon in the bottom right corner of the screen.

■ PLANNING CARE

After assessing your patient, you must begin the careful process of deciding what diagnoses best describe his or her condition. For each diagnosis, you will list outcomes that you want your patient to achieve. Then, based on each outcome, you will select nursing interventions that you believe will help your patient achieve the outcomes you selected. *Virtual Clinical Excursions—General Hospital* helps you in this process by providing a set of Planning Care resources. While you are still signed in for Elizabeth Washington, click on **Planning Care** in the upper left corner of the Nurses' Station screen. You will see two options: **Problem Identification** and **Setting Priorities**.

◆ Developing Nursing Diagnoses

Click on **Problem Identification**, and a note from your preceptor appears offering guidance about Ms. Washington's problems and possible diagnoses for the types of problems she may have. This diagnosis list is based on what expert nurses believe are *possible* for this particular patient. Remember, however, that not all of the diagnoses listed may apply to your patient—and that your patient may have other diagnoses that are not on the list. Your challenge and responsibility is to decide what nursing diagnoses *do* apply to your patient during each period of care. Since your patient's condition may be changing, some diagnoses may apply in one period of care but not in another. Read over the list of possible diagnoses for Elizabeth Washington. When you are finished, click on **Nurses' Station** to close the Problem Identification note.

Click again on **Planning Care**. This time select **Setting Priorities**. This will open another note from your preceptor. Notice that in the third paragraph of the note, your preceptor instructs you to use the Nursing Care Matrix. This is a resource designed to help you develop nursing diagnoses for your patient. To see how this resource works, click on the **Nursing Care Matrix** button at the bottom of the screen. Before you can develop nursing diagnoses, you must be sure your patient actually has the characteristics of those diagnoses. It is nearly impossible for anyone to remember all of the defining characteristics for every diagnosis, so nurses consult references such as *Nursing Diagnoses: Definitions and Classification, 2001–2002* (NANDA, 2001). To make your life a little simpler and to provide training in the health informatics resources of the future, the Nursing Care Matrix provides a list of diagnoses common for your type of patient, as well as the definition for each diagnosis and the defining characteristics for each diagnosis. Ackley and Ladwig (*Nursing Diagnosis Handbook: A Guide to Planning Care*, 5th edition) have mapped specific NANDA diagnoses onto major health-illness transitions. This mapping, along with input from our expert panel of nurses, provided the list of diagnoses you see—nursing diagnoses that *might* apply to Elizabeth Washington.

- Click on the first diagnosis. Note that the definition for this diagnosis now appears in a box in the upper right of the screen. The defining characteristics are listed in the box in the lower right of the screen.
- Click on another diagnosis. Review the definition and characteristics.

◆ Developing Outcomes and Interventions

For every nursing diagnosis you make, you can then select appropriate outcomes that you want your patient to achieve.

- Click on a diagnosis.
- Now click on **Outcomes and Interventions** at the bottom of the screen.
- On the left-hand side of the screen, you should now see the diagnosis you selected, along with a list of the outcomes you may want your patient to achieve if she has this diagnosis.

These outcomes are based on *Nursing Outcomes Classification*, 2nd edition (Johnson, Maas, and Moorhead, 2000). This reference provides detailed lists of linkages between the NANDA diagnoses and nursing outcomes defined in the *Nursing Outcomes Classification*.

For each outcome listed, you can access a list of nursing interventions to help your patient achieve that outcome.

- Click on the first outcome listed.
- On the right side of your screen, you will now see lists of intervention labels in three boxes: Major Interventions, Suggested Interventions, and Optional Interventions.

Each of the intervention labels in these boxes refers to an intervention that could be implemented to help achieve the specific outcome chosen. The *Nursing Intervention Classification* system gives a label to each intervention. Therefore, the Major, Suggested, and Optional Interventions are labels, each of which has a set of nursing activities that together comprise an intervention. If you look up a label in the *Nursing Interventions Classification*, you will see that it refers to a set of different nursing activities, some or all of which can be implemented in order to achieve the desired patient outcome for that diagnosis. We used *Nursing Diagnoses, Outcomes, and Interventions: NANDA, NOC and NIC Linkages* (Johnson, Bulechek, McCloskey-Dochterman, Mass, and Moorhead, 2001) and the *Nursing Interventions Classification*, 3rd edition, (McCloskey and Bulechek, 2000) to create the linkages between outcomes and interventions shown in the Nursing Care Matrix.

The Nursing Care Matrix provides you with a basic framework for learning how to move from making a diagnosis to defining patient outcomes and then to choosing the interventions you should implement to achieve those outcomes. Your instructor and the exercises in this workbook will help you develop this part of the nursing process and will provide you with more information about the nursing activities that belong with each intervention label.

■ CLINICAL REVIEW

Virtual Clinical Excursions—General Hospital also incorporates a learning assessment system called the Clinical Review, which provides quizzes that evaluate your knowledge of your patient's condition and related conditions.

- If you are still in the Nursing Care Matrix, return to the Nurses' Station by clicking first on **Return to Diagnoses** at the bottom of the Outcomes and Interventions screen and then on **Return to Nurses' Station** at the bottom of the Diagnosis screen.
- From the menu options in the upper left corner, click on **Clinical Review**.
- You will now see a warning box that asks you to confirm that you wish to continue. Click **Clinical Review Center**.

You are now looking at the opening screen for the Clinical Review Center. You have three quiz options: **Safe Practice**, **Nursing Diagnoses**, and **Clinical Judgment**. Do not click on any quiz buttons yet. First, read the following descriptions of the quizzes you can select:

- **Safe Practice**
  The **Safe Practice** quiz presents you with NCLEX-type questions based on the patient you worked with during this period of care. A set of five questions is randomly drawn from a pool of questions. Answer the questions, and the Clinical Review Center will score your performance.

- **Nursing Diagnoses**
  If you click on the **Nursing Diagnoses** button, you are presented with a list of 20 NANDA nursing diagnoses. You must select the five diagnoses in this list that most likely apply to your patient. The Clinical Review Center records your choices, gathers those choices that are correct, and scores your performance. The quiz then allows you to select nursing interventions for each of the outcomes associated with NANDA diagnoses that your correctly chose. For each of your correct diagnoses, you are presented with the likely outcomes for that diagnosis; for each outcome, you will see a list of six

nursing intervention labels. Only three of the intervention labels are appropriate for each outcome. You must select the correct labels. Again, your performance is automatically scored.

- **Clinical Judgment**
  The **Clinical Judgment** quiz asks you to consider a single question. This question evaluates your understanding of your patient's condition during the period of care in which you have just worked. Select your answer from four options related to your perception of your patient's stability and the frequency of monitoring you should be conducting.

You can take one, two, or all three of the quizzes. On any floor, when you are done with the quizzes, you must click on **Finish**. This will take you to a **Preceptor's Evaluation**, which offers a scorecard of your performance on the quizzes, discusses your understanding of the patient's condition and related conditions, and makes recommendations for you to improve your understanding.

Preceptor's Evaluation

Clinical Review

	Correct Responses	Score
Safe Practice	3.0	18.0
Implementing Nursing Care	4.0	16.0
Clinical Judgment	1.0	20.0
Totals		54.0
Total Score	Out of 100 possible points, you received 54.0 points or 54.0%	

Preceptor's Evaluation of Clinical Review

Clincial Judgment Recommendation - Congratulations! You made a good clinical decision about your client during this period of care

We want you to spend time practicing questions like those found in the Safe Practice assessment. These questions are very similar to those found on the NCLEX-RN. Also, we feel you need to study the nursing diagnoses approved by the North American Nursing Diagnosis Association (NANDA). Importantly, we want you to review the outcomes appropriate for a particular diagnosis as well as the interventions you would implement to achieve each outcome. You might want to spend time re-examining the diagnoses-outcomes-interventions linkages found in the Nursing Care Matrix. As mentioned above, the nursing diagnoses are based on approved diagnoses of the North American Nursing Diagnosis Association (NANDA). Remember that the outcomes are based on the Nursing Outcomes Classification and the interventions are based on the Nursing Interventions Classification (NIC).

Print a detailed report | Nurses' Station

Note: We don't recommend that you take any quizzes before working with a patient. The goal of *Virtual Clinical Excursions—General Hospital* is to help you learn and prepare for practice as a professional nurse. Reading your textbook, using this workbook to complete the CD-ROM activities, and organizing your thoughts about your patient's condition will help you prepare for the quizzes. More important, this work will help you prepare for care of real-life patients in clinical settings.

■ HOW TO QUIT OR CHANGE PATIENTS

Eventually, you will want to take a short or long break, begin caring for a different patient, or exit the software.

◆ To Take a Short Break

- Go to the Nurses' Station.
- Click on **Leave the Floor**, an icon in the lower left corner of the screen.
- You will see a screen with a variety of options.
- Click on **Break** and you will be given a 10-minute break. This stops the clock. After 10 minutes you are automatically returned to the floor, where you reenter the simulation at the same moment in time that you left.

◆ To Change Patients

Choose option 1 or option 2 below, depending on which activities you have completed during this period of care.

1. Use the following instructions *if you have already completed one or more of the quizzes* in the Clinical Review Center for your current patient:

   - Double-click on the **Supervisor's (Login) Computer** in the Nurses' Station.
   - Read the instructions for logging in for a new patient and period of care.
   - If you want to select a new patient on the *same* floor, click **Login**, select the new patient and period of care, and then click **Nurses' Station**.
   - If you want to work with a patient on a *different* floor, click **Return to Nurses' Station**, take the elevator to the new floor, and sign in for the new patient on the Login computer in the Nurses' Station.

2. Use the following instructions *if you have not completed any of the quizzes* in the Clinical Review Center for your current patient:

   - Double-click on the **Supervisor's (Login) Computer** in the Nurses' Station.
   - Read the instructions in the Warning box. Then click on **Supervisor's Computer**.
   - The computer logs you off and gives you the option of going to the Clinical Review Center or to the Nurses' Station. Unless you wish to go to the Clinical Review Center for evaluation of the period of care you just completed, click on **Nurses' Station**.
   - Double-click on the **Login Computer** again, and follow the instructions to sign in for another patient. (See the third and fourth bullets in option 1 above for specific steps.)

When you visit the patients on the Pediatric Floor (Floor 3), you will need to swap disks by following these steps:

- If up are currently signed in for a patient, go to the Supervisor's (Login) Computer and sign out. Return to the Nurses' Station.

- Leave the Nurses' Station and enter the elevator. Once you are inside the elevator, remove the disk from your CD-ROM drive and replace it with the other disk.

- Click on the button of the floor number where you need to go.

◆ **To Quit the Software for a Long Break or to Reset a Simulation**

- From the Nurses' Station, click on **Leave the Floor** in the lower left corner of the screen.
- You will see a new screen with a variety of options.
- You may select Quit with Bookmark or Quit with Reset.
  - **Quit with Bookmark** allows you to leave the simulation and return at the same virtual time you left. Any data you entered in the EPR will remain intact. Choose this option if you want to stop working for more than 10 minutes but wish to reenter the floor later at the exact point at which you left.
  - **Quit with Reset** allows you to quit and reset the simulation. This option erases any data you entered in the EPR during your current session. Choose this option if you know you will be starting a new simulation when you return.

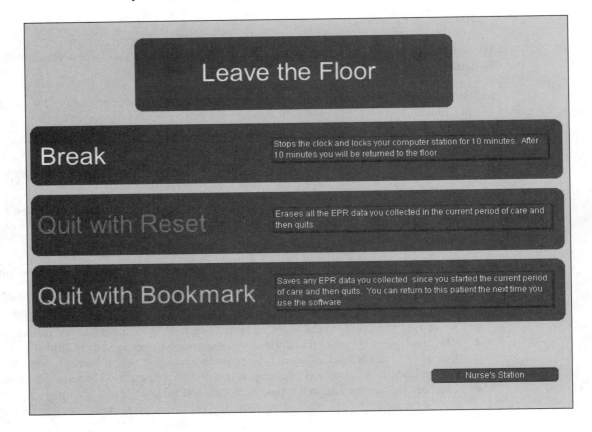

◆ **To Practice Exiting the Software**

- Click **Leave the Floor**.
- Now click **Quit with Reset**.
- A small message box will appear to confirm that you wish to quit and erase any data collected or recorded.
  - If you have reached this message in error, click the red X in the upper right corner to close this box. You may now choose one of the other options for leaving the floor (Break or Quit with Bookmark).
  - If you *do* wish to Quit with Reset, click **OK** on the message box.
- *Virtual Clinical Excursions—General Hospital* will close, and you will be returned to your computer's desktop screen.

A DETAILED TOUR

What do you experience when you care for patients during a clinical rotation? Well, you may be assigned one or several patients that need your attention. You follow the nursing process, assessing your patients, diagnosing each patient's problems or areas of concern, planning their care and setting outcomes you hope they will achieve, implementing care based on the outcomes you have set, and then evaluating the outcomes of your care. It is important to remember that the nursing process is not a static, one-time series of steps. Instead, you loop through the process again and again, continually assessing your patient, reaffirming your earlier diagnoses and perhaps finding improvement in some areas and new problems in other areas, adjusting your plan of care, implementing care as planned or implementing a revised plan, and evaluating patient outcomes to decide whether your patients are achieving expected outcomes. Patient care is hands-on, action-packed, often complex, and sometimes frightening. You must be prepared and present—physically, intellectually, and emotionally.

Textbooks help you build a foundation of knowledge about patient care. Clinical rotations help you apply and extend that book-based learning to the real world. You will know this with certainty when you experience it yourself—for example, when you first read about starting an IV but then have to start an IV on an actual patient, or when you read about the adverse effects of a medication and you then observe these adverse effects emerging in a patient. Stepping from a book onto a hospital floor seems difficult and unsettling. *Virtual Clinical Excursions—General Hospital* is designed as an intermediate tool to help you make the transition from book-based learning to the real world of patient care. The CD-ROM activities provide you with the practice necessary to make that transition by letting you apply your book-based knowledge to virtual patients in simulated settings and situations. Each simulation was developed by an expert nurse or nurse-physician team and is based on realistic patient problems, with a rich variety of data that can be collected during assessment of the patient.

Several types of patient records are available for you to access and analyze. This workbook, the software, and your textbook work together to allow you to move from ***book-based learning*** to real-life ***problem-based learning***. Your foundational knowledge is based on what you have learned from the textbook. The *VCE—General Hospital* patient simulations allow you to explore this knowledge in the context of a virtual hospital with virtual patients. Questions stimulated by the software can be answered by consulting your textbook or reviewing a patient simulation. The workbook is similar to a map or guide, providing a means of connecting textbook content to the practice of skills, data collection, and data interpretation by leading you through a variety of relevant activities based on simulated patients' conditions.

To better understand how *Virtual Clinical Excursions—General Hospital* can help you in your transition, take the following detailed tour, in which you visit three different patients.

■ WORKING WITH A MEDICAL-SURGICAL FLOOR PATIENT

In *Virtual Clinical Excursions—General Hospital*, the Pediatric Floor, the Intensive Care Unit, and Medical-Surgical/Telemetry Floor can be visited between 07:00 and 15:00, but you can care for only one patient at a time and only in the following blocks of time, which we call *periods of care*: 07:00–08:29, 09:00–10:29, 11:00–12:29, and 13:00–14:29. For each clinical simulation, you will select a single patient and a period of care. When you have completed the assigned care for that patient, you can then select a new patient and period of care. You can also reset a simulation at any point and work through the same period of care as many times as you want. Each time you sign in for a patient and time period, you will enter that session at the beginning of that period of care (unless you have previously "saved" a session by choosing Break or Quit with Bookmark).

Consider, for a moment, a typical Intesive Care Unit during the period between 07:00 and 15:00. Suppose that you could accompany a preceptor on that floor and provide care for patients during that 8-hour shift. Different expert nurses might take slightly different approaches, but almost certainly each nurse would establish priorities for patient care. These priorities would be based on report during shift change, a review of the patient records, and the nurse's own assessment of each patient.

At the beginning of a period of care, the assessment of each patient is usually accomplished by a general survey, that is, a fairly complete assessment of a patient's physical and psychosocial status. After the general survey, a nurse subsequently conducts focused assessments during the rest of the shift. The specific types of data collected in such focused assessments are determined by the nurse's interpretation of each patient's condition, needs, and applicable clinical pathways for independent and collaborative care. Depending on an agency's protocols and standards of care for the ICU patient, a nurse may conduct more than one comprehensive assessment during a shift, with focused surveys completed between the general surveys. Regardless of individual agency protocol, any ICU patient would have at least one general survey and numerous focused surveys over the period of the shift.

Now let's put these guidelines to practice by entering the ICU (Disk 2) at Canyon View Regional Medical Center. This time, you will care for James Story, a 42-year-old male suffering from renal failure.

1. **Enter and Sign In for James Story**

   - Insert your *VCE—General Hospital* Disk 2 in your CD-ROM drive and double-click on the **VCE—General Hospital** icon on your desktop. Wait for the program to load.
   - When Canyon View Regional Medical Center appears on your screen, click on the hospital entrance to enter the lobby.
   - Click on the elevator. Once inside, click on the panel to the right of the door; then click on button **5** for the Intensive Care Unit (ICU).
   - When the elevator opens onto the Intensive Care Unit, click on the **Nurses' Station**.
   - Inside the Nurses' Station, double-click on the **Supervisor's (Login) Computer** and select James Story as your patient for the 09:00–10:29 period of care.

2. **Case Overview**

   - Signing in automatically takes you to the patient's Case Overview. Your preceptor will appear and speak briefly on the video screen.
   - Listen to the preceptor; then click on **Assignment** below the video screen.
   - You will now see a Preceptor Note, which is a summary of care for James Story, covering the period of care just before the one you are now working.
   - Review the summary of care. Scroll down to read the entire report.
   - On the next page, make note of any information that you feel is important or that will require follow-up work, either with the patient or through examination of his records.

Areas of Concern for James Story:

- When you have finished the case overview, click on **Nurses' Station** in the lower right corner of the screen and you will find yourself in the ICU Nurses' Station.

3. Initial Impressions

Visit your patient immediately to get an initial impression of his condition.

- On the menu in the upper left corner of your screen, click on **Patient Care**. From the options on the drop-down menu, click on **Data Collection**. *Remember:* You can also visit the patient by double-clicking on the door to his room (Room 512).
- In the anteroom, wash your hands by double-clicking on the sink. Then click on the curtain to enter the patient area.
- Inside the room, you will see many different options for assessing this patient. First, click on **Initial Observations** in the top left corner of the screen. Observe and listen to the interaction between the nurse preceptor and the patient. Note any areas of concern, issues, or assessments that you may want to pursue later.
- Now that you have gotten an initial impression of your patient, you have a few choices. In some cases, you might wish to leave the patient and access his records to develop a better understanding of his condition and what has happened since he was admitted. However, let's stay with Mr. Story a while longer to conduct a few physical and psychosocial assessments.

4. Vital Signs

Obtain a full set of vital signs from James Story.

- Click on **Vital Signs** (just below the Initial Observations button). This activates a pathway that allows you to measure all or just some of your patient's vital signs. Four options now appear under the picture of James Story. Clicking on any of these options will begin a data collection sequence (usually a short video) in which the respective vital sign is measured. The vital signs data change over time to reflect the temporal changes you would find in a patient such as Mr. Story. Try the various vital signs options to see what kinds of data are obtained.
  - First, click on **BP/SpO$_2$/HR**. Wait for the video to begin; then observe as the nurse preceptor uses a noninvasive monitor to measure Mr. Story's blood pressure, SpO$_2$, and heart rate. After the video stops, the preceptor's findings appear as digital readings on a monitor to the right of the video screen. Record these data in the chart below. If you want to replay the video, simply click again on **BP/SpO$_2$/HR**. *Note:* You can replay any video in this manner—as often as needed.
  - Now click on **Respiratory Rate**. This time, after the video plays, an image of a breathing body model appears on the right. Count the respirations for the amount of time recommended by your instructor. Record your measurement below.
  - Next, click on **Temperature**. Again, a video shows the nurse preceptor obtaining this vital sign, and the result is shown on a close-up of a digital thermometer on the right side of the screen. Record this finding in the chart below.
  - Finally, click on **Pain Assessment** and observe as the nurse preceptor asks Mr. Story about his pain. Note Mr. Story's response in the chart below.

Vital Signs	Time
Blood pressure	
SpO$_2$	
Heart rate	
Respiratory rate	
Temperature	
Pain rating	

5. Mental Status

From some of your vital signs assessments, you should be starting to form an idea of Mr. Story's mental status. However, you can check his mental status more specifically by doing the following:

- On the left side of the Data Collection screen is a body model. When you move your cursor along the body, it begins to rotate and the area beneath your cursor is highlighted in orange.
- Place your cursor on the head area of the body model and click.
- Notice that new assessment options now appear under the picture of your patient.
- Click on **Mental Status** (the bottom option of the list).
- Observe Mr. Story's responses and interactions with the nurse. Then review the data, if any, that appear to the right after the video has stopped.

6. Respiratory Assessment

Auscultate Mr. Story's lungs to see whether there is any evidence of adventitious lung sounds.

- Click on the chest area of the body model.
- Note the new assessment options that come up beneath the picture of Mr. Story.
- Click on **Respiratory**.
- Observe the examination of the anterior, lateral, and posterior chest. Then review the data collected by your preceptor.
- Do you believe there is any evidence of problems? If so, explain what data support your conclusion.
- If you were worried about potential problems, what other assessments might you conduct?

7. Behavior

Since this is your first visit with Mr. Story, you may also want to collect some psychosocial data.

- At the bottom left corner of the screen, click on **Behavior**.
- One at a time, click on each of the behavioral assessment options that appear below the picture of Mr. Story.
- As you observe each assessment, take notes on the nurse-patient interactions.
- Do any of his responses concern you?
- Does he have family support as well as nursing support?
- What other questions do you want to ask Mr. Story? When might you ask these questions?

8. Chart

You have conducted your preliminary examination of James Story. Next, review his patient records.

- To access the patient Charts, either click on the stack of charts inside the Nurses' Station or click on **Patient Records** and then **Chart** from the drop-down menu.
- James Story's Chart automatically appears since you are signed in to care for him. As described earlier in **A Quick Tour**, the Chart is divided into several sections. Each section is marked by a colored tab at the bottom of the screen. To flip forward and back through the Chart sections, click on the labeled tabs and on the **Flip Back** icon, respectively. Once you have moved beyond a section, the tab for that section disappears. You can move back to previous sections *only* by clicking on the **Flip Back** icon, which appears above the Nurses' Station icon in the lower right corner.

- Review the following sections of Mr. Story's chart: History & Physical, Nursing History, Operative Reports, and Progress Notes.
- Based on your analyses of these records and your preliminary assessment of Mr. Story, summarize key issues for this patient's care in the box below.
- When you are finished, close the chart by clicking on the **Nurses' Station** icon.

Key Issues for Patient Care:

---

9. Electronic Patient Record (EPR)

Now examine the data in James Story's EPR.

- To access the EPR, first click **Patient Records** in the upper left corner of the screen. Then click **EPR** on the drop-down menu. *Remember:* As an alternative, you can also double-click on the EPR computer in the Nurses' Station. This computer is located to the left of the Kardex and has **Electronic Patient Records** on the screen.
- On the EPR access screen, enter the password—**nurse2b**—and click **Access Records**.
- The EPR automatically opens to the patient's Vital Signs summary. Examine James Story's vital signs data for the past 8 hours.
- Now click **Respiratory** (three buttons below Vital Signs). The data from assessments of Mr. Story's respiratory system are now shown.
- Examine Mr. Story's data. Record your findings in the box on the next page.

Lung Sounds During the Past 24 Hours:

- Next, click on **Cardiovascular**.
- Review data collected for edema.
- List any evidence for fluid retention as evidenced by edema.
- If edema was observed, make sure you note the location(s) and quality.
- Note any other data that indicate problems.
- Now, make an assessment of Mr. Story's clinical status:

Cardiovascular Data:

a. Are any of the vital signs data you collected this morning significantly different from the baselines for those vital signs?

Circle One: Yes   No

b. If "Yes," which data are different?

c. Do you have any concerns about the data collected during your respiratory assessment?

Circle One: Yes   No

d. If you answered "No," what data tell you the patient is stable?

e. If you answered "Yes," what are your concerns?

10. Medication Administration Record (MAR)

- James Story has been taking a number of medications. Access his current MAR by double-clicking on the notebook below the MAR sign in the Nurse' Station. You can also open the MAR by clicking on **Patient Records** and then on **MAR** on the drop-down menu.
- Once the MAR notebook is open, access Mr. Story's records by clicking on the tab with his room number (512) at the bottom of the screen.
- Examine the MAR and note any medications that Mr. Story should be given during the period of care between 09:00 and 10:29. Make a list of these medications, the times they are to be administered, and any assessments you should conduct before and after giving the medications.

Medication Data:

- Click the **Nurses' Station** icon to close the MAR.

11. Planning Care

So far, you have completed a preliminary examination of James Story and reviewed some of his records. Now you can begin to plan his care. *Note:* Before *actually* starting a plan of care, you would conduct a more thorough assessment and a more complete review of this patient's records. However, let's continue so that you can learn how to use *Virtual Clinical Excursion's* unique and valuable Planning Care resource.

- On the drop-down menu, click **Planning Care** and then **Problem Identification**.
- Read the Preceptor Note for James Story and write one nursing diagnosis that you think might apply to this patient. Base your decision on your preliminary assessment and review of his records.

Nursing Diagnosis:

- Click on **Nurses' Station** to close this note.
- Click again on **Planning Care** in the upper left corner of your screen. This time, select **Setting Priorities** from the drop-down menu.
- Review the Preceptor Note on setting priorities for James Story.
- When you have finished, click on **Nursing Care Matrix** at the bottom of your screen.
- You will now see a list of nursing diagnoses approved by the North American Nursing Diagnosis Association (NANDA) that may apply to Mr. Story's condition.
- Find the diagnosis you just identified for Mr. Story. Click on this diagnosis.

- Review the nursing diagnosis definition and the defining characteristics that now appear on the right side of the screen.
- Does the definition fit your patient?
- Does your patient have the defining characteristics? If not, perhaps your assessment was not complete enough for you to make this decision. What other assessments should you conduct in order to determine whether this diagnosis applies to James Story?
- For now, assume that your diagnosis *does* apply to Mr. Story. Click on the **Outcomes and Interventions** button at the bottom of the screen.
- You now see a screen that lists nursing outcomes for your diagnosis. These are based on the Nursing Outcomes Classification. If your patient has this diagnosis, these are the outcomes you will want him to achieve.
- Some or all of these outcomes will probably apply to your patient if he does indeed have the nursing diagnosis you selected.
- Click on the first outcome, and text will appear in the three boxes on the right side of the screen. These boxes show the Major, Suggested, and Optional Interventions that could be implemented to achieve the outcome you selected, based on the Nursing Interventions Classification. *Remember:* Each entry listed in these boxes is an intervention label that represents a *set* of nursing activities that you would implement.
- Review the nursing interventions, especially those in the Major Interventions box. These are the most likely interventions you would implement to achieve the outcome you have clicked. However, you should consider all of the interventions before deciding which apply to the outcome for your patient.
- Now click on **Return to Diagnoses**. At this time, you can explore other diagnoses and their respective outcomes and interventions, or you can click **Return to Nurses' Station**.

Your work with James Story is completed for now. To quit the software and reset a simulation:

- Go to the Nurses' Station.
- Click on **Leave the Floor** in the lower left corner of the screen.
- A screen appears with a variety of options.
- Select **Quit with Reset**, which allows you to quit and reset the simulation. This option erases any data you entered in the EPR during your current session.

■ WORKING WITH A PERIOPERATIVE PATIENT

One of the patients at Canyon View Regional Medical Center, Darlene Martin, has been admitted to undergo a total abdominal hysterectomy.

- In the Surgery Department (Disk 2) on Floor 4, sign in to visit Darlene Martin for her Preoperative Interview.
- After viewing the Case Overview and reading the Assignment, return to the Nurses' Station. Click on **Patient Care** and then **Data Collection** on the drop-down menu.
- Wash your hands, enter the room, and click **View Interview**.
- After observing the interview, click on **Summary** and read the Preceptor Note.
- Now return to the Nurses' Station and sign out of this period of care.
- Click on the **Supervisor's (Login) Computer** again and sign in to visit Ms. Martin during her preoperative care.
- Although you cannot observe Ms. Martin's surgery, you can see her now in the Preoperative Care Bay and later in the PACU
- Once Ms. Martin is transferred out of PACU, you can visit her in her room on the Medical-Surgical/Telemetry Floor (Floor 6).

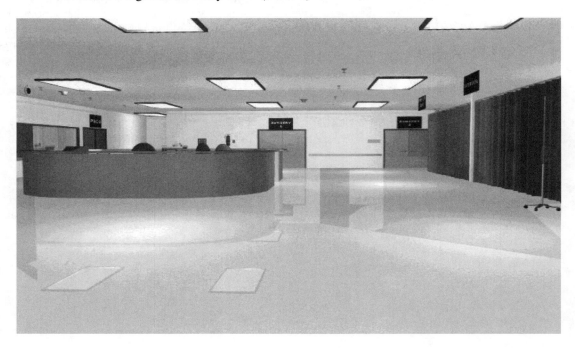

- Spend some time in each of the different perioperative settings in the Surgery Department, as described on p. 38. Then compare these perioperative settings with the settings on the Pediatric Floor and the Medical-Surgical/Telemetry Floor. Use the following chart and focus your comparisons on the themes listed in the left column.

Comparison of Settings in Canyon View Regional Medical Center			
Activities and Resources	Perioperative Settings	Pediatric Floor Settings	Medical-Surgical/ Telemetry Floor Settings
Patient Assessments			
Planning Care			
Types of Patient Records			

Remember: *Virtual Clinical Excursions—General Hospital* is designed to provide a realistic learning environment. Within Canyon View Regional Medical Center, you will not necessarily find the same type of patient records, clinical settings, Nurses' Station layout, or hospital floor architecture that you find in your real-life clinical rotations. If you have already had experience within actual clinical settings, take a few moments to list the similarities and differences between the Canyon View virtual hospital and the real hospitals you have visited. There is considerable variation among hospitals in the United States, so think of *Virtual Clinical Excursions—General Hospital* as simply one type of hospital and take advantage of the opportunity to practice learning how, where, when, and why to find the information, medication, and equipment resources you need to provide the highest quality patient care.

The following icons are used throughout the workbook to help you quickly identify particular activities and assignments:

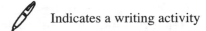 Indicates a reading assignment—tells you which textbook chapter(s) you should read before starting each lesson

Indicates a writing activity

Marks the beginning of an interactive CD-ROM activity—signals you to open or return to your *Virtual Clinical Excursions—General Hospital* CD-ROM

Indicates a continuation of CD-ROM activity instructions

Indicates questions and activities that require you to consult your textbook

LESSON **1** _____

Coordinating Patient Care— Part 1

_____

Client Need Categories: Nursing Process, Communication, and Documentation

Reading Assignment: Physical Assessment (Chapter 4)
Nursing Process and Critical Thinking (Chapter 5)
Documentation (Chapter 6)

Patient: Elizabeth Washington, Room 604

Objectives

1. After doing a data collection, record important information that will facilitate nursing care for your patient.
2. Determine whether your patient has an advance directive and what actions you will need to take secondary to this determination.
3. Review the patient's chart to acquire needed information in order to determine appropriate care.
4. Review physician orders to determine what consultations with other health care team members have been ordered.
5. Determine whether services that have been ordered by other members of the health care team have been provided and whether they meet the patient's needs.
6. Identify what actions you will need to take to coordinate care with the patient's family.
7. Determine independent and collaborative care after reviewing the physician's order.
8. Determine the sequence of patient care for the first $1\frac{1}{2}$ hours of your assignment for this patient.

Introduction

Physical and emotional safety of the patient is the responsibility of the nurse. The following lesson will assist you in determining appropriate actions to provide care for your patient's needs. In order to coordinate care with other health care team members, the nurse must collaborate with staff, physicians, family, and members of other departments. The LPN/LVN usually coordinates care on the unit assigned under the RN's direction with other staff and physicians.

Decisions about patient care are also the responsibility of the nurse. The LPN/LVN makes patient care decisions about expected and common procedures for which guidelines are provided. Any unusual orders are handled by the RN, who also does the scheduling and establishes new sequences of activities for patient care. This lesson will assist you in making appropriate decisions about the coordination of patient care.

CD-ROM Activity

Insert *Virtual Clinical Excursions—General Hospital* Disk 2 in your CD-ROM drive and click on the **Shortcut to VCE** icon on your computer's desktop. Enter the hospital by clicking on the front doors. Once inside the lobby, click on the elevator and go to the Medical-Surgical/Telemetry Floor (Floor 6). When you arrive on the floor, click on the **Nurses' Station**; then double-click on the **Supervisor's (Login) Computer**. Sign in to work with Elizabeth Washington in Room 604 for the 07:00–08:29 period of care. Listen to the Case Overview, click on **Assignment**, and read the Preceptor Note.

1. Complete the following form as you read the Preceptor Note. Record vital information that will assist you in providing care for Ms. Washington.

Patient's Name	Age	Diagnosis
Medical History	Surgery	Current Medications
Assessment Information	IV	Wound/Dressing
Activity and Positioning	Other Pertinent Information	

2. What information would be helpful but was not provided by the Preceptor Notes? (*Hint:* Refer to Physical Assessment Guide on p. 61 of your textbook.)

3. Based on the information that you have recorded in questions 1 and 2, list at least five assessments that you will need to make upon entering Ms. Washington's room. (*Hint:* Refer to pp. 60–70 of your textbook.)

   a.

   b.

   c.

   d.

   e.

Now that you have received the report from your preceptor, it is time to go to your patient's room and perform a data collection. Return to the Nurses' Station, click on **Patient Care**, and choose **Data Collection** from the drop-down menu. Don't forget to wash your hands by double-clicking on the sink. Double-click on the curtain to enter Ms. Washington's room. Click on **Initial Observations** and listen to a short conversation between the nurse and patient. Then click on the various buttons and parts of the body model on the left and observe the nurse carrying out the physical assessment of Ms. Washington. When additional assessment options appear under the video screen, click on each button to gather specific data. (*Note:* You will record your findings in the following questions.)

4. Below, take notes that will assist you in planning your care and developing priorities by recording the data you collected from the physical assessment. Place an asterisk (*) next to any findings that are abnormal. (*Hint:* For more information on initial assessments, see Chapter 4 of your textbook.)

Blood pressure

SpO$_2$

Heart rate

Respiration

Temperature

Pain

IV

Wound

Nutrition

Behavior

Other data gathered

Now, determine the status of your patient by answering the following questions.

5. Is Ms. Washington having any symptoms because of her medical problems? If so, what are her symptoms, and what action should you take?

6. Based on your findings in question 4, are Ms. Washington's vital signs stable? If not, what actions are required?

7. Do any other findings from the Data Collection indicate that you need to take further action? If so, what action is needed?

8. What is the status of your patient? Write a statement about Ms. Washington's condition.

→ Return to the Nurses' Station, click on **Patient Records**, and choose **Chart** from the drop-down menu. Review Ms. Washington's Chart to acquire more information and determine appropriate care for her. To go forward through the sections of the Chart, click on the tabs at the bottom of the screen. To move backward to previous sections, click on the **Flip Back** icon until you have reached the desired record. (*Note:* To move back and forth through the pages *within* a section of the Chart, you may use the scroll bar on the right side of the Chart or the page number arrows on the lower left corner of the Chart.)

9. Provide the following information from the History & Physical section of Ms. Washington's Chart.

   a. Impression of the Emergency Department physician:

   b. Plan as determined by ED physician:

   c. Results from the diagnostic tests done in the ED (*Hint:* See the first page of the History & Physical, the Emergency Department Record):

   d. Treatment Ms. Washington received in ED:

→ Return to the Nurses' Station and click on **Case Conference**. One at a time, select the choices in the drop-down menu and review the explanations of Independent Care and Collaborative Care. Based on your review, determine which current orders you can initiate by yourself (independent care) and which ones you will need to coordinate with other health care team members (collaborative care).

10. In your own words, explain and differentiate between independent care and collaborative care. (*Hint:* Refer to pp. 80–81 of your textbook for more information.)

→ Now that you know what types of care are possible, return to the Nurses' Station. Click on **Patient Records** and review Ms. Washington's Chart and Kardex.

11. Below, list examples of dependent and collaborative care you found for Ms. Washington. Identify whether you found each example in the patient's Chart or in the Kardex.

Dependent care

Collaborative care

12. Several orders need to be carried out during your assigned time with Ms. Washington. You will need to prioritize the orders to determine what nursing actions are needed. List those actions in chronological order below.

13. Below, chart all of the actions you listed in question 13. Follow the recommended charting rules found in your textbook. (*Hint:* See p. 98 of your textbook for more information.)

In this section you will determine whether services that have been ordered by the physician have been provided and, if not, what action you will need to take to ensure that Ms. Washington's needs are met.

Return to the Nurses' Station, click on **Patient Records**, and choose **Chart** from the drop-down menu. Click on the **Physician Orders** tab and search for any services/consults ordered for Ms. Washington.

14. List any services that have been ordered by the physician. Then check to see whether the services have been initiated. (*Hint:* Click on the **Consults** tab.) If you find a record that indicates the service has been provided, list the results below. If you cannot find a record documenting the service provided, indicate what action you would initiate.

15. Consult a drug reference and complete the following table to become familiar with enoxarin.

Enoxarin

Uses   Recommended doses and route

Side effects   Cautions

Contraindications

16. One of the physician orders on Tuesday at 06:30 is to teach the patient/family how to administer enoxarin SQ. What actions will you need to take in order to ensure that this is done and that the patient and family understand the procedure and can administer the drug safely?

Ask your instructor whether you should complete the Clinical Review. If so, proceed with that review. If not, quit the program by following the directions given in the **Getting Started** section of this book.

2

Coordinating Patient Care— Part 2

Client Need Categories: Patient's Rights, Confidentiality, Advocacy, and Continuity of Care

Reading Assignment: Legal and Ethical Aspects of Nursing (Chapter 2)
Communication (Chapter 3)

Patient: Elizabeth Washington, Room 604

Objectives

1. Use communication techniques that will promote a trusting relationship with your patient.
2. Determine appropriate actions that will protect your patient's information and records.
3. Use ethical practices to protect your patient from invasion of privacy.
4. Review preoperative physician orders and patient records to determine whether the patient was informed of the impressions of the physician and the recommended plan of care.
5. Investigate the preoperative checklist to determine what actions were taken to inform the family and patient about patient responsibilities and self-care before surgery.
6. Discuss the actions, documentation, and communication needed to promote continuity of care for the patient between preoperative, intraoperative, and postoperative care.

Introduction

Maintaining the patient's rights and confidentiality and being an advocate for the patient are some of the duties of the LPN/LVN. All information about the patient should be released only to other health care team members directly providing care for the patient. The patient has rights to make decisions regarding her care, to have health care provided without any prejudice, and to be treated with dignity and respect at all times. The nurse must understand these rights and be willing to be the patient's advocate to ensure they are not violated. This lesson will assist you in determining appropriate actions to help you to maintain your responsibilities regarding patient rights, confidentiality, informed consent, advocacy, and understanding ethical practices. Decisions about who may have access to patient's records and information must be made by the nurse to ensure the patient's privacy. The concept of caring and cultural awareness must also be integrated into your patient care. This lesson will assist you in maintaining a caring, supportive atmosphere for your patient while protecting her rights.

CD-ROM Activity

Insert *Virtual Clinical Excursions—General Hospital* Disk 2 in your CD-ROM drive and click on the **Shortcut to VCE** icon on your computer's desktop. Enter the hospital by clicking on the front doors. Once inside the lobby, click on the elevator and go to the Medical-Surgical/Telemetry Floor (Floor 6). When you arrive on the floor, click on the **Nurses' Station**, then double-click on the **Supervisor's (Login) Computer**. Sign in to work with Elizabeth Washington in Room 604 for the11:00–12:29 period of care. Listen to the Case Overview, click on **Assignment**, and read the Preceptor Note before returning to the Nurses' Station.

Part of establishing a trusting relationship with your patient is basic communication. In the upper left corner of the Nurses' Station screen, click on **Patient Care** and choose **Data Collection** from the drop-down menu. (*Remember:* This takes you to the sink area outside the patient's room. You must wash your hands and click on the curtain before you are allowed to enter the room.) Since the initial assessment of this patient was done earlier in the day, you will need to focus on other assessments. Click on **Behavior** and then select **Signs of Distress** from the list below the video screen. Listen to the conversation between the nurse and Ms. Washington and then answer the following question.

 1. List the nonverbal cues of communication used by the nurse during the Signs of Distress assessment. (*Hint:* See pp. 31–32 in your textbook for cues.)

Nonverbal Cues	Changes in Communication You Would Make (If Any)
Voice	
Eye contact	
Physical appearance	
Gestures	
Posture	

→ Click on **Needs** and then on **Support**. While listening to the conversations, note the verbal therapeutic communication techniques and answer the questions below.

   2. List an example for each of the following:

An open-ended question

A closed-ended question

A clarifying statement

   3. During the Data Collection, you should have observed the nurse and Ms. Washington discussing the use of the call light. (*Hint:* To review this interaction, return to Ms. Washington's room; then click on **Behavior** and select **Needs** from the center menu.) Based on your observation of the nurse in the video, what would you do differently to make sure that Ms. Washington understands how to use the call light?

→ Now that you have ensured that Ms. Washington is able to call for help, return to the Nurses' Station.

   4. Often when a patient is involved in an auto accident, there is an investigation. You have just left your patient's room and notice that someone in the Nurses' Station is looking at your patient's Chart, which you left lying on the counter. This person is not wearing a uniform and does not have an official name tag. You have never seen him before. Determine appropriate actions that will protect your patient's information and records. What action would you take and why?

   5. The man says that he is an attorney and that you should mind your own business. What action will you take next?

6. The man still refuses to do as you ask. What will you do now?

7. The man tells you that you will be charged with interfering with an investigation. How would you respond to this?

8. What would you do now that the man knows Ms. Washington's room number?

➤ From the Nurses' Station, click on **Patient Records** and select **Chart** from the drop-down menu. Review the History & Physical, Physician Orders, and Operative Reports sections to answer the following questions.

9. Review the preoperative physician orders and determine whether the patient was informed of the impressions of the physician and the recommended plan of care. What was the recommendation for care? Where in Ms. Washington's Chart did you find this information?

10. Investigate the preoperative checklist to determine what actions were taken to inform family and patient about patient responsibilities and self-care before surgery. (*Hint:* See Operative Reports.) List the actions that were taken and documented on the preoperative patient instruction sheet. (*Hint:* Also in Operative Reports section.) This sheet illustrates that the patient and family were informed about exactly what was going to happen and what the patient and family could do to ensure that the patient was ready for surgery.

11. There are three phases of any surgical procedure: preoperative (before surgery), intraoperative (during surgery), and postoperative (after surgery). Return to the Operative Reports section of Ms. Washington's Chart and find all three of these phases illustrating how the health care team documented communication or actions that promoted continuity of care. List examples of each phase below. Discuss the actions, documentation, and communication needed to promote continuity of care for the patient between preoperative, intraoperative, and postoperative care. (*Note:* If you have not studied these phases of surgery, review the information about informed consent. The focus of this assignment is to discuss communication of information in the Chart. At the bottom of the chart below, list any other statements that you find helpful to promote continuity of care.)

Preoperative	Intraoperative	Postoperative

Safety and Infection Control—Part 1

Client Need Categories: Medical and Surgical Asepsis and Standard/Universal and Other Precautions

Reading Assignment: Medical/Surgical Asepsis and Infection Control (Chapter 12)

Patient: Elizabeth Washington, Room 604

Objectives

1. Check your patient's areas for possible sources of infection.
2. Correctly perform aseptic techniques.
3. Apply principles of infection control.
4. Identify modes of organism transmission.
5. Monitor the use of infection control precautions by other staff members.
6. Identify signs of wound infection.
7. Discuss appropriate infection control procedures with your patient and family.

Introduction

A patient who has entered a health care facility has a higher chance of exposure to disease-causing organisms. The nurse must be able to identify and report symptoms of any infectious processes. For a patient who has had damage to the skin, which is the first line of defense, the need for infection control principles and procedures is of utmost importance. Therefore, medical and surgical asepsis maintenance must become a part of the nurse's practice to provide a safe and effective care environment with the control of infections executed in every action of every nurse.

Decisions about what procedures to follow, when to use precautions, and how to identify signs of infections will be explored in this lesson. You will need to determine what actions to take to ensure an environment that will minimize your patient's risk for development of an infectious process.

CD-ROM Activity

Insert *Virtual Clinical Excursions—General Hospital* Disk 2 in your CD-ROM drive and click on the **Shortcut to VCE** icon on your computer's desktop. Enter the hospital by clicking on the front doors. Once inside the lobby, click on the elevator and go to the Medical-Surgical/Telemetry Floor (Floor 6). When you arrive on the floor, click on the **Nurses' Station**; then double-click on the **Supervisor's (Login) Computer**. Sign in to work with Elizabeth Washington in Room 604 for the period of 09:00–10:29. Listen to the Case Overview, click on **Assignment**, and read the Preceptor's Note before returning to the Nurses' Station.

In the upper left corner of the Nurses' Station screen, click on **Patient Care** and choose **Data Collection** from the drop-down menu. (*Remember:* This takes you to the sink area outside the patient's room. You must wash your hands before you are allowed to enter the room.) In Ms. Washington's case, the body's first line of defense has been damaged as a result of hip surgery, so it is now necessary to assess how well she is handling this break in her skin integrity. Click on **Wound Condition**. Observe the nurse's assessment of the wound and then answer the following question about Ms. Washington's wound.

1. What steps did the nurse take to be able to see the patient's wound?

 2. Refer to your textbook and review the principles of infection control. List them below and circle the principles of infection control that the nurse used with Ms. Washington. Briefly explain why the nurse used the principles you circled. (*Hint:* See pp. 236, 241, and 242 of your textbook.)

3. Why did the nurse touch the skin along the wound? (*Hint:* See Inflammatory Response on p. 238 of your textbook for more information.)

4. Why did the nurse ask Ms. Washington whether she was having any tenderness?

5. What specific techniques of assessment must you use to determine whether a patient with dark skin color has redness?

6. What should the wound look like if it is healing properly?

→ Return to the Nurses' Station, click on **Patient Records**, and choose **EPR** from the drop-down menu. (*Remember:* To enter the EPR, you must type the password—**nurse2b**—and then click on **Access Records**.) Inside the EPR, click on **Wounds and Dressings** and review the most recent data documented under "Appearance," "Drainage," and "Dressing."

7. Several different findings are documented in Ms. Washington's EPR. Explain why each of the normal findings listed below is significant. Also identify what significance the findings would have if they were abnormal.

Normal Assessment	Significance	Abnormal Significance
Left hip surgical incision is well approximated and open to air		
No drainage from site		
No redness around edges		

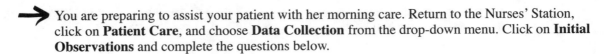

You are preparing to assist your patient with her morning care. Return to the Nurses' Station, click on **Patient Care**, and choose **Data Collection** from the drop-down menu. Click on **Initial Observations** and complete the questions below.

8. Identify factors of the patient environment that you can control to protect Ms. Washington from a nosocomial infection.

 9. List the modes of organism transmission. (*Hint:* Refer to p. 237 of your textbook.)

Continue your Data Collection by clicking on the various buttons and parts of the body model on the left side of the screen. Watch for modes of organism transmission.

10. Do you see any modes of organism transmission present in your patient's environment? If so, what action do you need to take to prevent transmission of infection?

11. What activities of assisting your patient with her morning care would increase her chances of being exposed to infectious organisms?

12. An assistant is helping you with Ms. Washington's care, and you notice that she enters the room and begins to empty the trash. After she has done this, she lays linen on the sink top and begins to prepare the basin of water for Ms. Washington's bath. What important principle of infection control did the assistant forget to do? What action should you take?

13. Ms. Washington will need to be told how to take care of her wound after her discharge. What directions can you give her to help her in prevention of a wound infection? If you are not familiar with the proper care for a wound, refer to your textbook and explain how you would ensure that the patient knows how to do the care.

14. Ms. Washington's husband is also present in the room. What will you need to tell him about prevention of infection in the home after his wife's discharge from the hospital?

Safety and Infection Control—Part 2

Client Need Categories: Handling Hazardous and Infectious Materials,
Use of Restraints, and Disaster Planning

Reading Assignment: Safety (Chapter 13)

Patients: Elizabeth Washington, Room 604

Objectives

1. Assist in adapting home environment to meet your patient's safety needs.
2. Follow a nursing care plan to assist your patient in meeting safety needs related to her fractured hip and prescribed treatments.
3. Provide safe use of equipment such as oxygen, mobility aids and safety devices.
4. Check with your patient to ensure correct use of safety devices for increased mobility and improved motor skills.
5. Review medication orders for completeness.
6. Protect your patient from injury.

Introduction

When a patient enters a health care facility, the nurse must be able to provide an environment that is free from dangers due to falls, electrical hazards, fires, burns, and poisoning. The responsibility for providing and maintaining a safe environment is always within the nurse's role; therefore protecting the patient from injury, as well as patient education, must be included in the daily care of the patient. Upon discharge, the patient will need to know how to adjust her home environment to accommodate the new mobility restrictions. As a nurse, you must be alert and aware of potential situations that may harm the patient or the patient's family members, as well as yourself. This lesson will explore potential safety hazards and direct your actions for prevention of injury.

CD-ROM Activity

Insert *Virtual Clinical Excursions—General Hospital* Disk 2 in your CD-ROM drive and click on the **Shortcut to VCE** icon on your computer's desktop. Enter the hospital by clicking on the front doors. Once inside the lobby, click on the elevator and go to the Medical-Surgical/Telemetry Floor (Floor 6). When you arrive on the floor, click on the **Nurses' Station**; then double-click on the **Supervisor's (Login) Computer**. Sign in to work with Elizabeth Washington in Room 604 for the 09:00–10:29 period of care. Listen to the Case Overview, click on **Assignment**, and read the Preceptor Note before returning to the Nurses' Station. From the Nurses' Station, click on **Planning Care** and choose **Problem Identification** from the drop-down menu.

1. As you prepare to assist Ms. Washington in ambulation, you will need to follow the nursing care plan to ensure her safety. List the nursing diagnoses that have been identified by the RN.

2. Which of the diagnoses will apply only to the perioperative area? Why?

→ Return to the Nurses' Station, click on **Planning Care**, and choose **Setting Priorities** from the drop-down menu. At the bottom of your screen, below the Preceptor Note, click on the button labeled **Nursing Care Matrix**. This reference lists the possible nursing diagnoses for Ms. Washington. Clicking on a diagnosis reveals the definition and characteristics for that diagnosis.

3. From the list on the left side of the screen, select the nursing diagnoses that are related to mobility. List those diagnoses below and on the next page. For each diagnosis, provide the definition and characteristics.

Nursing Diagnosis	Definition	Characteristics

Nursing Diagnosis	Definition	Characteristics

4. In the first column below and on the next page, rewrite the nursing diagnoses you identified in question 3. For each diagnosis, identify the expected outcome for Ms. Washington. Then provide major interventions, as well as suggested and optional interventions, to achieve each outcome. Be sure to list any assistive devices that will be required for her mobility.

Nursing Diagnosis	Expected Outcome	Major Interventions	Suggested and Optional Interventions

Nursing Diagnosis	Expected Outcome	Major Interventions	Suggested and Optional Interventions

5. Any time that a patient has to learn to move again after a trauma, the nurse must be cautious. Ms. Washington's ability to walk as she did before the accident has been altered. List what safety principles you will need to employ to ensure that your patient will not fall while learning to walk after this injury. (*Hint:* To review safety in the health care environment and older adult considerations, refer to p. 270 of your textbook.)

6. Below, list precautions that promote safety. Circle the ones that apply specifically to Ms. Washington.

7. List questions that you could ask Ms. Washington about her home environment to assist her in realizing what changes will have to be made to alleviate accident potentials. (*Hint:* See "Safety Promotion" on p. 275 of your textbook or for more information.)

8. What patient teaching will you have to provide your patient and family to ensure that there will not be an accident after she is discharged and returns home?

→ Return to the Nurses' Station, click on **Patient Records**, and choose **Chart** from the drop-down menu. Within the Chart, click on **Medication Records** and review the medications Ms. Washington is receiving.

9. Below and on the next page, list the medications that Ms. Washington is receiving. Next, identify three common side effects of each medication. Complete the table below by explaining what effect each medication may have on her ability to move about safely. (*Hint:* You may need to consult a drug reference to complete this exercise.)

Medications and Strength	Side Effects	Possible Effect on Mobility

Medications and Strength	Side Effects	Possible Effect on Mobility

LESSON **5** —————————————————————

Growth and Development Through the Life Span— Part 1

Client Need Categories: Aging Process, Family Interaction Patterns, and Developmental Stages and Transitions

Reading Assignment: Health Promotion for the Infant, Child, and Adolescent (Chapter 28)
Basic Pediatric Nursing Care (Chapter 29)
Care of the Child with a Physical Disorder (Chapter 30)

Patient: Maria Ortiz, Room 308

Objectives

1. Assist your patient with developmental transition.
2. Assist your patient in choosing age-appropriate recreational activities, considering her preferences and physical capabilities.
3. Compare your patient's psychosocial, behavioral, and physical development with norms for her age and developmental stage.
4. Consider age and developmental stage when discussing procedures or surgery with your patient.
5. Monitor your patient's achievement of appropriate developmental levels.
6. Provide physical care appropriate to the developmental level of your patient.
7. Provide age-appropriate activities to your patient according to developmental norms.

Introduction

Health care for the pediatric patient focuses on fostering health promotion through health supervision and health maintenance, including processes such as immunization, screenings, and surveillance. However, when the patient is acutely ill, management of the patient and her condition become quite different. The nurse needs to be able to provide care for the child while also supporting the family. The family must be involved in all care decisions and assist with care as appropriate. This lesson presents situations that will assist you in the development of supportive techniques to deal with the special psychosocial and physical changes that a pediatric patient and her family experience during an acute illness.

CD-ROM Activity

Insert *Virtual Clinical Excursions—General Hospital* Disk 2 in your CD-ROM drive and click on the **Shortcut to VCE** icon on your computer's desktop. Enter the hospital by clicking on the front doors. Once inside the lobby, click on the elevator, and go to the Pediatric Floor (Floor 3).

When you arrive at the floor, click on the **Nurses' Station**; double-click on the **Supervisor's (Login) Computer** and sign in to work with Maria Ortiz in Room 308 for the 07:00–08:29 period of care. Listen to the Case Overview, click on **Assignment**, and read the Preceptor Note before returning to the Nurses' Station. In the upper left corner of the Nurses' Station screen, click on **Patient Care** and choose **Data Collection** from the drop-down menu. (*Remember:* This takes you to the sink area outside the patient's room. You must wash your hands before you are allowed to enter the room.) Inside the patient's room, click on the various buttons and parts of the body model on the left side of the screen and observe the nurse carrying out the physical assessment of Maria Ortiz. (*Note:* Record your findings in question 1.)

 1. Review the data collection of Maria Ortiz and document your findings on the chart below and on the next two pages. (*Note:* Be sure to write as if you were documenting directly in your patient's Chart.) In the right column, identify whether each finding is normal or abnormal. List the significance of any abnormal findings. (*Hint:* Refer to Chapter 29 of your textbook for more information.)

Assessment	Findings	Normal or Abnormal? (list significance if abnormal)
Initial Observations		
Vital Signs Blood pressure		
SpO$_2$		
Heart rate		
Respiration		
Temperature		
Pain Assessment		
Head & Neck		
Chest & Back		
Upper Extremities		

Assessment	Findings	Normal or Abnormal? (list significance if abnormal)
Lower Extremities		
GI & GU		
Perineum & Rectum		
IV		
Nutrition Oral		
Parenteral		
Output		

Assessment	Findings	Normal or Abnormal? (list significance if abnormal)
Behavior Signs of Distress		
Needs		
Support		
Understanding		
Activity		

→ Leave Maria's room by clicking on Nurses' Station in the lower right hand corner of your screen. This will take you back to the sink area; wash your hands again and double-click on the door to return to the Nurses' Station.

Maria has had asthma for some time now and has been admitted to the Emergency Department twice before this episode. She may be experiencing psychosocial and behavioral development problems. Click on **Patient Records** and choose **Chart** from the drop-down menu.

 2. Spend the next few minutes reviewing Maria's entire Chart. Below and on the next page, make notes that will assist you in determining age-appropriate activities for Maria. Keep in mind that activities will include nursing care, as well as activities that are important to Maria and that will help her in play and socialization. (*Hint:* For ideas on what notes to take, refer to Chapter 29 of your textbook.)

Patient Record	Notes
History & Physical	
Nursing History	
Admissions Records	
Physician Orders	
Progress Records	
Laboratory Reports	

Patient Record	Notes

X-Rays & Diagnostics

Medication Records

 3. In the left column below, identify Maria's developmental stage and list behaviors that are appropriate for her age group. In the right column, list behaviors that you noticed during your observation of Maria that could indicate she is not adjusting to her disease process. (*Hint:* Refresh your memory of the Data Collection on Maria by rereading your findings in question 1. See p. 799 of your textbook as a reference.)

Developmental Stage and Appropriate Behaviors for an 8-Year-Old	What Evidence Could Indicate That Maria Is Not Adjusting?

Return to the Nurses' Station, click on **Planning Care**, and choose **Problem Identification** from the drop-down menu. Of the diagnoses listed as possibilities, select six that deal with Maria's physical capabilities and list them in the left column of question 4 on the next page. Now return to the Nurses' Station, click on **Planning Care**, and choose **Setting Priorities** from the drop-down menu. At the bottom of your screen, below the Preceptor Note, click on the button labeled **Nursing Care Matrix**. In the left-hand column, find and click on the first diagnosis you listed for Maria in question 4 and read its definition and characteristics. Then click on the **Outcomes and Interventions** button at the bottom of the screen. Next, select an outcome for the diagnosis you have chosen. Identify appropriate interventions for Maria from the lists on the right side of the screen. List your chosen outcomes and interventions in the appropriate columns of the table in question 4. Finally, provide a rationale for each intervention. Continue this process for each diagnosis in your list.

4. Use the table below to record appropriate nursing diagnoses, outcomes, interventions, and rationales for Maria. (*Hint*: See instructions on previous page.)

Nursing Diagnosis	Expected Outcomes	Interventions	Rationale

Since Maria's mother is present and is supporting Maria during this hospitalization, it is the responsibility of the nurse to assess the level of adjustment that she is making to her daughter's illness. Return to the Nurses' Station, click on **Planning Care**, and select **Problem Identification**. Identify nursing diagnoses that may be appropriate for Ms. Ortiz. Once again, return to the Nurses' Station and click on **Planning Care**. Select **Setting Priorities** and then click on the **Nursing Care Matrix** button. From the list of nursing diagnoses, select those that deal with Maria's mother's adjustment. For each diagnosis you choose, read the definition and characteristics. Then click on **Outcomes and Interventions** and choose expected outcomes and interventions.

5. Below, list appropriate nursing diagnoses for Maria's mother. For each diagnosis, state the expected outcome and identify interventions to achieve that outcome. Provide a rationale for each intervention. (*Hint:* See Chapter 29 of your textbook for help.)

Nursing Diagnosis	Expected Outcome	Interventions	Rationale

6. Refer to the care plan you completed and your notes above to determine additional age-appropriate activities you can implement for Maria. List them below and provide a rationale for each activity.

Activities	Rationale

Growth and Development Through the Life Span— Part 2

Client Need Categories: Human Sexuality and Expected Body Image Changes
Reading Assignment: Health Promotion for the Infant, Child, and Adolescent
(Chapter 28)
Basic Pediatric Nursing Care (Chapter 29)
Care of the Child with a Physical Disorder (Chapter 30)

Patient: De Olp, Room 310

Objectives

1. Monitor the impact of expected body image changes on your patient and family.
2. Monitor your patient's reaction to age-related changes.
3. Identify expected physiologic changes according to your patient's age.
4. Suggest modified approaches for providing care in accordance with your patient's developmental stage.
5. Assist in referring your patient and family to resources necessary to maintain or promote appropriate family functioning.
6. Identify the family structure and roles of family members.
7. Monitor stressors that may have an impact on family functioning.
8. Promote appropriate parental roles.

Introduction

The diagnosis of cancer in children is a catastrophic, highly emotional, and life-altering experience for the child and the family. The patient's reaction to the disease and the changes that will occur because of the disease and its treatment need to be closely watched and managed. The LPN/LVN must be alert not only to physical changes but also to the emotional responses to the newly diagnosed disease. This lesson will allow you to investigate the physiologic changes and to support the patient and the family as they respond physically and emotionally to this life-changing situation.

CD-ROM Activity

Insert *Virtual Clinical Excursions—General Hospital* Disk 2 in your CD-ROM drive and click on the **Shortcut to VCE** icon on your computer's desktop. Enter the hospital by clicking on the front doors. Once inside the lobby, proceed to the elevator and go to the Pediatric Floor (Floor 3). When you arrive at the floor, click on the **Nurses' Station**; then double-click on the **Supervisor's (Login) Computer** and sign in to work with De Olp in Room 310 for the 07:00–08:29

period of care. Listen to the Case Overview, click on **Assignment**, and read the Preceptor Note before returning to the Nurses' Station.

1. Complete the form below with information from the Case Overview and Preceptor Note.

Patient's Name	Age	Diagnosis
Medical History	Surgery/Procedures Lumbar Puncture	Current Medications
		Last pain med
Assessment Information	IV	Wound/Dressing
Activity and Positioning	Other Pertinent Information (i.e., lab results)	

2. De Olp has been newly diagnosed with acute lymphoblastic leukemia (ALL). Referring to p. 831 of your textbook, complete the short information data sheet below and on the next page as a review of this condition. (*Hint:* Use a medical dictionary or reference book to investigate any words you are not familiar with.)

Definition of leukemia

Etiology/pathophysiology

Clinical manifestations

Diagnostics tests

Medical management

Nursing interventions

Patient teaching

Prognosis

→ Return to the Nurses' Station, click on **Patient Records**, and choose **Chart** from the drop-down menu. Review De's History & Physical and Nursing History to gain a better understanding of her current physical condition as it relates to her medical diagnosis. This information can also be found in her Electronic Patient Record (EPR). To access that record, return to the Nurses' Station, click on **Patient Care**, and choose **EPR**. Enter the password—**nurse2b**—and click **Access Records**.

3. Find the areas of these records showing physical changes that may be occurring in De and complete the table below.

Assessment Area	Data That Document Physical Changes
Vital Signs	
Neurologic	
Musculoskeletal & Neck	

Assessment Area	Data That Document Physical Changes
Cardiovascular	
GI & GU	
Wounds	
Safety & Comfort	
Behavior & Activity	

→ Return to the Nurses' Station, click on **Planning Care**, and choose **Problem Identification** from the drop-down menu. Read the Preceptor Note. Find the list of possible nursing diagnoses for De and record these in the table for question 4. Return to the Nurses' Station, click on **Planning Care**, and choose **Setting Priorities** from the drop-down menu. Click on **Nursing Care Matrix** at the bottom of the Setting Priorities screen. In the left-hand column of the screen, find and select the first nursing diagnosis on your list. After reading the definition and characteristics of the diagnosis, click on **Outcomes and Interventions** at the bottom of the screen. Next, select an expected outcome for the diagnosis and identify appropriate interventions. List your chosen outcome and interventions in the corresponding columns of the table in question 4. Finally, provide a rationale for each intervention. Continue this process for each diagnosis in your list.

4. Use the table below to record appropriate nursing diagnoses, outcomes, and interventions for De. (*Hint*: See Planning Care instructions on previous page.) Be sure to provide a rationale for each intervention listed.

Nursing Diagnosis	Expected Outcomes	Interventions	Rationale

→ De's father is present and will need emotional support and patient teaching. Return to the Nurses' Station, click on **Patient Care**, and choose **Data Collection** from the drop-down menu. Click on the **Behavior** button on the left.

5. Collect and record data about De's behavior below. Include De's father's remarks and concerns. (*Hint:* See pp. 797-803 of your textbook for reference.)

Signs of Distress

Needs

Support

Understanding

Activity

6. What stressors will affect the family's functioning? (*Hint:* See p. 802 of your textbook for Factors Affecting Parents' Reactions.)

7. How can you assist the family in maintaining appropriate family roles?

8. What referrals can you make that will support the reduction of the stressors and maintain appropriate family roles?

LESSON 7

Prevention and Early Detection of Disease— Part 1

Client Need Categories: Data Collection Techniques, Health Screening, and Immunizations

Reading Assignment: Physical Assessment (Chapter 4)

Health Promotion for the Infant, Child, and Adolescent (Chapter 28)

Care of the Child with a Physical Disorder (Chapter 30)

Patient: De Olp, Room 310

Objectives

1. Document expected and abnormal findings noted on physical examination of your patient.
2. Use general principles that will reinforce your patient and family teaching.
3. Perform aspects of a data collection during a physical examination of your patient.
4. Prepare your patient for a physical examination.
5. Report physical examination results to health care team members and document findings.
6. Review your patient's and her family's understanding of health risks and promotion.

Introduction

The nurse must be able to identify conditions that may cause the patient's condition to worsen. Health promotion and adjustments to a disease process should focus on lifestyle practices that will promote continued wellness for the patient. Being able to assist the patient and family in health promotion is important. This lesson will direct you through data collection during a physical assessment of the pediatric patient, including the determination of the patient's ability for self-care. The family will be encouraged to participate in the patient's care and wellness promotion.

CD-ROM Activity

Insert *Virtual Clinical Excursions—General Hospital* Disk 2 in your CD-ROM drive and click on the **Shortcut to VCE** icon on your computer's desktop. Enter the hospital by clicking on the front doors. Once inside the lobby, click on the elevator and go to the Pediatric Floor (Floor 3). When you arrive at the floor, click on the **Nurses' Station**; then double-click on the **Supervisor's (Login) Computer**. Sign in to work with De Olp in Room 310 for the 07:00–08:29 period of care. Listen to the Case Overview, click on **Assignment**, and read the Preceptor Note before returning to the Nurses' Station. Then click on **Patient Care** and choose **Data Collection** from the drop-down menu. Inside the patient's room, click on the various buttons and parts of the body model on the left and observe the nurse carrying out the physical examination of De Olp. As you proceed, record your findings in question 1.

1. Complete the data assessment of De Olp and document your findings on the chart below and on the next two pages. In the right column identify whether each finding is normal or abnormal. List the significance of any abnormal findings.

Assessment	Findings	Normal or Abnormal (list significance if abnormal)
Initial Observations		
Vital Signs		
Blood pressure		
SpO$_2$		
Heart rate		
Respiration		
Temperature		
Pain Assessment		
Head & Neck		
Chest & Back		
Upper Extremities		
Lower Extremities		

Assessment	Findings	Normal or Abnormal (list significance if abnormal)
GI & GU		
Perineum & Rectum		
IV		
Wound Condition		
Nutrition Oral		
Parenteral		
Output		

Assessment	Findings	Normal or Abnormal (list significance if abnormal)
Behavior		
Signs of Distress		
Needs		
Support		
Understanding		
Activity		

2. Which of your findings will need attention or nursing interventions?

3. During your data collection, De mentions that she was scared before the lumbar puncture. What nursing interventions could you have done if you had been the nurse preparing De and her father for this diagnostic test? If you are not familiar with the lumbar puncture procedure, consult your medical dictionary or another reference book. (*Hint:* For helpful information, also see p. 808 of your textbook.)

4. If you had to prepare a teaching tool that would help you tell De about the placement of the Port-o-Cath, what would you prepare? Describe your teaching plan and list any tools or materials you would need. (*Hint:* See p. 801 of your textbook for suggested interventions for Age-Related Fears Associated with Surgery.)

5. What communication techniques should you use?

6. What should you tell De's father about the procedure?

7. Is there anything else you could do to prepare De for this procedure?

8. During your data collection De mentions that the doctor said that she had something wrong with her blood. Would you explain to her the risks of the disease and what precautions she would need to take? Do you think she is ready for this information? If so, why? If not, why not? (*Hint:* You may need to refer to reference material on leukemia.)

9. What specific information will De's father need about leukemia? Do you think he is ready for this information? If so, why? If not, why not?

Prevention and Early Detection of Disease— Part 2

Client Need Categories: Disease Prevention, Health Promotion Programs, and Lifestyle Choices

/OᴐꝹ **Reading Assignment:** Health Promotion for the Infant, Child, and Adolescent (Chapter 28)

Care of the Child with a Physical Disorder (Chapter 30)

Patient: Maria Ortiz, Room 308

Objectives

1. Incorporate patient teaching to ensure that your patient and family understand prevention of complications and maintenance of optimum health status.
2. Review your patient's and family's understanding of health risks and promotion.
3. Determine your patient's ability and support for performing self-care.
4. Assist your patient to accept the activity level demanded because of illness.
5. Assist your patent to maintain her level of self-care after unexpected body image changes.
6. Assist your patient to identify behaviors that could affect her health.
7. Encourage your patient to participate in behavior modification programs to promote health.
8. Review your patient's activities that could affect her health.

Introduction

The nurse must be able to identify conditions that may cause the patient's condition to worsen. Health promotion and adjustments to a disease process should focus on lifestyle activities that will promote continued wellness for the patient. Being able to monitor the physical and mental status of your patient will assist you in preventing complications and promoting an optimal level of wellness. In this lesson you will explore your patient's activities to promote her optimal level of wellness, including the determination of your patient's ability for self-care. The family will be encouraged to participate in the patient's care and wellness promotion.

CD-ROM Activity

Insert *Virtual Clinical Excursions—General Hospital* Disk 2 in your CD-ROM drive and click on the **Shortcut to VCE** icon on your computer's desktop. Enter the hospital by clicking on the front doors. Once inside the lobby, click on the elevator and go to the Pediatric Floor (Floor 3). When you arrive at the floor, click on the **Nurses' Station**; then double-click on the **Supervisor's (Login) Computer**. Sign in to work with Maria Ortiz in Room 308 for the 11:00–12:29 period of care. Listen to the Case Overview and read your Assignment before returning to the

Nurses' Station. In the upper left corner of the Nurses' Station screen, click on **Patient Care** and choose **Data Collection** from the drop-down menu. Click on the various buttons and parts of the body model on the left side of the screen and observe the nurse carrying out the physical assessment of Maria Ortiz. Record your findings in question 1.

1. Complete the assessment of Maria and document your findings on the chart below and on the next two pages. List the significance of each finding.

Assessment	Findings	Significance
Initial Observations		
Vital Signs		
Blood pressure		
SpO$_2$		
Heart rate		
Respiration		
Temperature		
Pain assessment		
Head & Neck		
Chest & Back		
Upper Extremities		

Assessment	Findings	Significances
Lower Extremities		
GI & GU		
Perineum & Rectum		
IV		
Nutrition Oral		
Parenteral		
Output		

Assessment	Findings	Significances
Behavior		
Signs of Distress		
Needs		
Support		
Understanding		
Activity		

2. Asthma is a condition that demands that the patient and family fully understand what they can do to help prevent attacks. As you should have noted in question 1, Maria has just had an episode of respiratory difficulty. What action should you take at this time? Why? (*Hint:* For more information on asthma, refer to pp. 842-844 of your textbook.)

During your assessment, you also should have noted the responses made by Maria's mother about her understanding of the disease process of asthma and how to prevent attacks. Review of the patient's and family's understanding can help keep Maria out of the hospital and help her prevent future asthma attacks. To incorporate patient teaching that will ensure Maria and her mother understand how to prevent attacks and the treatment of her condition, the nurse must plan and implement several different nursing actions.

→ Return to the Nurses' Station, click on **Planning Care**, and choose **Problem Identification** from the drop-down menu; then read the Preceptor Note. Return to the Nurses' Station, click on **Planning Care**, and choose **Setting Priorities**. At the bottom of your screen, below the Preceptor Note, click on the button labeled **Nursing Care Matrix**. Find the nursing diagnosis that pertains to compromised family coping (lack of knowledge). Once you select the appropriate nursing diagnosis, click on **Outcomes and Interventions**.

3. Below, modify the nursing diagnosis you chose so that you will know what definition, characteristics, outcome, and interventions will assist Maria and her mother in promoting optimal health status.

Definition

Characteristics

Outcome

Interventions

4. Maintaining comfort and self-care is part of Maria's planned care. Make a list of problems or situations that will interfere with Maria's ability to do self-care as a result of unexpected body image changes due to asthma attacks. (*Hint:* Access Maria's records, especially the Kardex, or refer to your textbook to locate likely problems or situations.)

5. For each problem or situation you listed in question 4, identify the nursing interventions that you could implement to support Maria in maintaining a level of self-care.

Problem/Situation   **Interventions**

6. Once Maria becomes more comfortable after this latest respiratory difficulty, what activities will she need to do to prevent another episode?

7. What things can Maria's mother do that will support the decrease of asthma attacks? What teaching can you provide?

8. What can you do to assist Maria and her mother to understand what activities will need to be done after discharge to prevent asthma attacks (and hospitalizations) in the future?

LESSON 9

Coping and Adaptation— Part 1

Client Need Categories: Coping Mechanisms, Religious and Spiritual Influences on Health, Situational Role Changes, End-of-Life Issues, and Grief and Loss

Reading Assignment: Communication (Chapter 3)
Basic Pediatric Nursing Care (Chapter 29)
Care of the Child with a Physical Disorder (Chapter 30)

Patient: De Olp, Room 310

Objectives

1. Discuss actions that will assist your patient and family cope with heath status.
2. Identify your patient's coping mechanisms.
3. Assist your patient and her family to find resources for coping with loss/bereavement.
4. Identify your patient's response to illness and compare with the normal patient's reaction.
5. Provide support to your patient with an altered body image.

Introduction

When children are experiencing difficult situations and illness, the nurse must provide support and assist the patient and family in coping with the illness. This support requires the nurse to be prepared for the situation and to establish a level of trust that will allow the patient and family to express their fears, apprehension, and anxiety. In this lesson you will investigate the development of this trusting relationship in order to assist your patient and her family to cope with the newly diagnosed illness.

CD-ROM Activity

Insert *Virtual Clinical Excursions—General Hospital* Disk 2 in your CD-ROM drive and click on the **Shortcut to VCE** icon on your computer's desktop. Enter the hospital by clicking on the front doors. Once inside the lobby, click on the elevator and go to the Pediatric Floor (Floor 3). When you arrive at the floor, click on the **Nurses' Station**; then double-click on the **Supervisor's (Login) Computer**. Sign in to work with De Olp in Room 310 for the 09:00–10:29 period of care. Listen to the Case Overview and read your Assignment before returning to the Nurses' Station.

Establishing a level of trust that will allow De and her father to talk with you about their fears and concerns can be accomplished during routine procedures and interventions. During the assessment of De at 09:00, you will have an opportunity to use communication to establish that relationship.

In the upper left corner of the Nurses' Station screen, click on **Patient Care** and choose **Data Collection** from the drop-down menu. Click on the various buttons and parts of the body model on the left and observe the nurse carrying out the physical assessment of De Olp.

 1. Complete the assessment of De and document your findings on the chart below and on the next page. Complete the right column by identifying communication that the nurse used or *could have used* to establish a trusting relationship. (*Hint:* See Chapter 29, p. 797, of your textbook for hints.)

Assessment	Findings	Communication the Nurse Used or Could Have Used to Establish a Trusting Relationship
Initial Observations		
Vital Signs Blood pressure		
SpO$_2$		
Heart rate		
Respiration		
Temperature		
Pain assessment		
IV		
Nutrition Oral		

Assessment	Findings	Communication the Nurse Used or Could Have Used to Establish a Trusting Relationship
Parenteral		
Output		
Behavior		
Signs of Distress		
Needs		
Support		
Understanding		
Activity		

Now that you have done a complete assessment of De, refer to Chapter 29 of your textbook for help with the following questions.

2. Since De is 6 years old, list specific developmental considerations/interventions that you will need to use when communicating with her. Be specific for her case.

3. While still referring to Chapter 29, list below any specific age-related concerns that De may have since she has been hospitalized. After you have listed the concerns, identify De's possible behaviors/responses and what actions you will want to take to support her in coping with the illness/hospitalization.

Concerns	Possible Behavior/ Responses by De	Nursing Actions

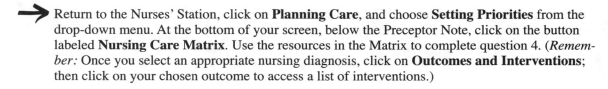 Return to the Nurses' Station, click on **Planning Care**, and choose **Setting Priorities** from the drop-down menu. At the bottom of your screen, below the Preceptor Note, click on the button labeled **Nursing Care Matrix**. Use the resources in the Matrix to complete question 4. (*Remember:* Once you select an appropriate nursing diagnosis, click on **Outcomes and Interventions**; then click on your chosen outcome to access a list of interventions.)

4. Since Mr. Olp is present with De and is supporting his daughter during this hospitalization, it is the responsibility of the nurse to assess the level of adjustment the patient and her father are making to this illness. Select the nursing diagnoses that deal with De's reactions, coping mechanisms, death anxiety, and self-image. List those diagnoses below and on the next page. For each diagnosis, list the definition, characteristics, outcome, and interventions that would be appropriate for De and her father. (*Note:* Your answers will vary depending on which diagnoses you select.)

Nursing Diagnosis	Definition	Characteristics	Outcome	Interventions

Nursing Diagnosis	Definition	Characteristics	Outcome	Interventions

Coping and Adaptation—
Part 2

Client Need Categories: Stress Management, Support Systems, Therapeutic
Communication, and Unexpected Body Image Changes

Reading Assignment: Cultural and Ethnic Considerations (Chapter 7)
Loss, Grief, Dying, and Death (Chapter 9)

Patient: James Story, Room 512

Objectives

1. Assist your patient to meet his spiritual needs.
2. Assist in evaluating whether the religious or spiritual needs of your patient are met.
3. Consider your patient's religious or spiritual beliefs in recommendations for the plan of care.
4. Help your patient adjust to change in roles.
5. Monitor your patient's and his family's abilities to adjust to changes in roles.
6. Recognize cultural differences in your patient's and his family members' roles.
7. Encourage your patient and his family to use stress management techniques.
8. Encourage your patient to use problem-solving skills using therapeutic communication techniques.
9. Implement measures to reduce environmental stressors for your patient.

Introduction

Chronic illness often causes your patient and patient's family to experience changes in roles, loss of independence, loss of the ability to support themselves, financially and physically, and a challenge to their ability to live without great stresses. The patient and family will have new spiritual, physical, and emotional needs. The nurse must be able to support the patient when spiritual needs influence health, when the patient experiences role changes, when end-of-life issues arise, and when grief and loss stress management becomes the major concern for the patient. This lesson directs you through the activities that will facilitate your ability to meet the demands of a patient who has a chronic illness that has affected his spiritual, physical, and mental well-being.

CD-ROM Activity

Insert _Virtual Clinical Excursions—General Hospital_ Disk 2 in your CD-ROM drive and click on the **Shortcut to VCE** icon on your computer's desktop. Once inside the lobby, click on the elevator, and go to the Intensive Care Unit (Floor 5). When you arrive at the floor, click on the **Nurses' Station**; then double-click on the **Supervisor's (Login) Computer**. Sign in to work with James Story in Room 512 for the 07:00–08:29 period of care. Listen to the Case Overview and read your Assignment before returning to the Nurses' Station. In the upper left corner of the Nurses' Station screen, click on **Patient Records** and choose **Chart** from the drop-down menu. In order to be able to support your patient, you must know as much as possible about him. Note taking will be a part of your care for patients. Develop a system that you can follow to become familiar with your patients. Be brief and specific. The object is not to rewrite the chart but to collect information that you can use in your patient's care.

1. Review James Story's Chart and complete the short note-taking table below and on the next page.

Chart Component	Notes	Why This Information is Important
History & Physical		
Nursing History		
Admissions Record		
Physician Orders		
Progress Notes		
Laboratory Reports		

Chart Component	Notes	Why This Information is Important
X-Rays & Diagnostics		
Operative Reports		
Medication Records		

In order to help your patient adjust to changes in roles, you must monitor his and his family's abilities to adjust to those changes. Now that you have an overall picture of Mr. Story's status, look at his emotional and spiritual state.

2. Referring to Mr. Story's Chart and the data that you recorded in question 1, list the times that Mr. Story or his wife mentioned his dissatisfaction with his current health status.

→ Return to the Nurses' Station, click on **Planning Care**, and choose **Problem Identification** from the drop-down menu. Read the Preceptor Note.

3. Review the nursing diagnoses in your textbook (p. 173) that relate to coping and adjustment, and the nursing diagnosis listed in the Problem Identification Preceptor Note. Decide which diagnoses you think best fit Mr. Story's and his wife's adjustment status and list them below.

4. Keeping Mr. Story's current physical status in mind, identify interventions that would be appropriate at this time for each diagnosis you listed in question 3. State your rationale for choosing these interventions. (*Remember:* Even though Mr. Story may not be dying at this moment, he and his wife are experiencing loss of a normal life.)

5. What interventions would be appropriate when Mr. Story is moved out of ICU once his condition stabilizes? Be sure to include measures that encourage him and his wife to use stress management and problem-solving techniques that will reduce environmental stressors during his illness. State your rationale for choosing these interventions.

6. Identify the spiritual and cultural influences that may affect Mr. Story in his adjustment to chronic illness and loss. (*Hint:* Refer to Chapter 7 of your textbook or any reference that presents information about spiritual beliefs.)

7. Describe any differences between your own cultural and spiritual beliefs and those of Mr. Story that may lead to incorrect assumptions about how Mr. Story is adjusting to his condition.

LESSON **11**

Basic Care and Comfort— Part 1

Client Need Categories: Nutrition, Oral Hydration, and Elimination
Reading Assignment: Selected Nursing Skills (Chapter 19)
Basic Nutrition and Nutritional Therapy (Chapter 20)
Fluids and Electrolytes (Chapter 21)

Patient: Paul Jungerson, Room 602

Objectives

1. Assist with teaching your patient about dietary modifications.
2. Monitor your patient's nutritional and hydration status.
3. Monitor your patient's hydration status.
4. Monitor your patient for the impact of his disease on his nutritional status.
5. Use measures to improve the nutritional intake for your patient.
6. Identify patient factors that could interfere with elimination.
7. Monitor your patient's elimination pattern and status.
8. Provide patient ostomy care.

Introduction

Patients with gastrointestinal disorders experience interference with normal intake and elimination that hampers their ability to maintain a consistent state of wellness. Inability to maintain nutritional status is a particularly common problem for a person who has had a colon resection and temporary colostomy. The disease process and its treatment can lead to severe protein-calorie malnutrition. Progressive wasting, weakness, debilitation, compromised immune function, potential therapy intolerance, and general poor health status may occur. This lesson will direct you through the assessment of your patient's nutritional status, hydration, and elimination patterns.

CD-ROM Activity

Insert *Virtual Clinical Excursions—General Hospital* Disk 2 in your CD-ROM drive and click on the **Shortcut to VCE** icon on your computer's desktop. Once inside the lobby, click on the elevator, and go to the Medical-Surgical/Telemetry Floor (Floor 6). When you arrive at the floor, click on the **Nurses' Station**; then double-click on the **Supervisor's (Login) Computer**. Sign in to work with Paul Jungerson in Room 310 for the 07:00–08:29 period of care. Listen to the Case Overview and read your Assignment before returning to the Nurses' Station. In the upper left corner of the Nurses' Station screen, click on **Patient Care** and choose **Data Collection** from the drop-down menu. Inside the patient's room, click on the various buttons and parts of the body model and observe the nurse carrying out the physical assessment of Mr. Jungerson.

1. Complete the short form below, based on the data you collected during Mr. Jungerson's physical assessment. The purpose of this form is to keep important notes to use as a reference during your care of the patient. Be as specific as you need, but don't write everything, since it is already recorded in the patient's chart.

Patient's Name	Age	Diagnosis
Medical History	Surgery	Current Medications Last pain med
Assessment Information	IV	Wound/Dressing
Activity and Positioning	Other Pertinent Information	

→ Return to the Nurses' Station, click on **Patient Records** and choose **EPR** from the drop-down menu to access the Electronic Patient Records. (*Remember:* If you prefer, you can double-click on the EPR computer on the counter in the Nurses' Station.) When prompted, type the password—**nurse2b**—and click **Access Records**.

2. Monitor the patient's nutritional and hydration status by completing the table below and on the next page. List data for Friday through Tuesday and the problems that you can identify based on the assessment of Mr. Jungerson's nutritional and hydration status. (*Note:* Information can be found in various parts of the patient's EPR and Chart.)

Diet on Friday

Diet	Diet intake	Intake (include IV)
Elimination	Bowel elimination	Weight
Skin turgor		

Diet on Saturday

Diet	Diet intake	Intake (include IV)
Elimination	Bowel elimination	Weight
Skin turgor		

Diet on Sunday

Diet	Diet Intake	Intake (include IV)
Elimination	Bowel elimination	Weight
Skin turgor		

Diet on Monday

Diet	Diet intake	Intake (include IV)
Elimination	Bowel elimination	Weight
Skin turgor		

Diet on Tuesday

Diet	Diet intake	Intake (include IV)
Elimination	Bowel elimination	Weight
Skin turgor		

Problems Because of Nutritional Status

3. The doctor has ordered a dietary consult for total parenteral nutrition (TPN). It will be your responsibility to assist in teaching the patient about TPN. Complete the exercise below by listing information that you would include in a teaching plan to help Mr. Jungerson understand the new dietary modifications. (*Hint:* Refer to Chapter 20 of your textbook for assistance).

Definition of total parenteral nutrition (TPN)

Why the doctor has ordered TPN

How this nutrition can be delivered

Advantages of PPN

Why TPN is indicated

Risk (state in terms the patient will understand, without increasing his anxiety)

→ Return to the Nurses' Station, click on **Planning Care**, and choose **Setting Priorities** from the drop-down menu. Click on **Nursing Care Matrix** at the bottom of the screen. From the list on the left part of the screen, find nursing diagnoses that address the problems you identified for Mr. Jungerson in question 2. (*Note:* List these in question 4 below.) Highlight one of your selected diagnoses; then click on **Outcomes and Interventions**. Now choose and click on the expected outcome most appropriate for Mr. Jungerson's problem. From the lists on the right, select interventions to achieve that outcome. After recording the outcome and interventions in question 4, click **Return to Diagnoses** to continue this process for each diagnosis you listed.

4. From the data that you gathered in question 2, list the status of your patient's elimination. What nursing interventions should you take to ensure elimination of bowel and urine?

Problem/ Nursing Diagnosis	Outcome	Interventions

→ Return to the Nurses' Station, click on **Patient Care**, and choose **Data Collection** from the drop-down menu. Click on **Nutrition** and then on **Output**.

5. During this data collection the nurse removes the colostomy bag. Notice the way the nurse removes the bag. List the needed equipment and steps you would take to provide ostomy care, replace the bag, and leave the patient comfortable. (*Hint:* Refer to Chapter 19 of your textbook for more information.) Be sure to write these steps in your own words to facilitate your mastery of the skill in clinical.

6. Below, complete an example Chart entry that shows the care you have just provided for Mr. Jungerson.

LESSON 12

Basic Care and Comfort—Part 2

Client Need Categories: Personal Hygiene

Reading Assignment: Hygiene and Care of the Patient's Environment (Chapter 17)

Patient: Paul Jungerson, Room 602

Objectives

1. Assist your patient to maintain or perform self-care.
2. Assist your patient in planning actions that support achievement of self-care needs.
3. Assist or provide your patient with basic hygiene and grooming.
4. Monitor your patient's ability to perform activities of daily living.
5. Reinforce patient teaching regarding required adaptation in the performance of activities of daily living.
6. Review usual personal hygiene habits and routines of your patient.

Introduction

Often patients are not capable of performing personal hygiene because of their condition and disease processes. The nurse's role is to assist the patient with personal care and promote medical asepsis and reduction of pathogens. This may involve doing all of the care for the patient, supporting the patient to do as much as possible, or assisting the patient to the shower or tub.

Activities of daily living (ADLs), comfort of environment, positioning, and prevention of skin breakdown are also important. The nurse must provide a safe, comfortable environment that will prevent skin breakdown and provide overall comfort. This lesson will direct you through the process of providing hygiene, maintaining skin integrity, and promoting comfortable surroundings.

CD-ROM Activity

Insert *Virtual Clinical Excursions—General Hospital* Disk 2 in your CD-ROM drive and click on the **Shortcut to VCE** icon on your computer's desktop. Enter the hospital by clicking on the front doors. Once inside the lobby, click on the elevator and go to the Medical-Surgical/Telemetry Floor (Floor 6). When you arrive at the floor, click on the **Nurses' Station**; then double-click on the **Supervisor's (Login) Computer**. Sign in to work with Paul Jungerson in Room 602 for the 09:00–10:29 period of care. Listen to the Case Overview and read your Assignment before returning to the Nurses' Station. In the upper left corner of the Nurses' Station screen, click on **Patient Care** and choose **Data Collection** from the drop-down menu. Click on the the various buttons and parts of the body model on the left to observe the nurse carrying out the physical assessment of Mr. Jungerson.

1. Complete the data collection of Mr. Jungerson and document your findings on the chart below and on the next two pages. Identify whether findings are normal or abnormal and list the significance of any abnormal findings.

Assessment	Findings	Normal or Abnormal? (list significances if abnormal)
Initial Observations		
Vital Signs		
Blood pressure		
SpO$_2$		
Heart rate		
Respiratory rate		
Temperature		
Pain assessment		
Head & Neck		
Chest & Back		
Upper Extremities		

Assessment	Findings	Normal or Abnormal? (list significances if abnormal)
Lower Extremities		
GI & GU		
Perineum & Rectum		
IV		
Wound Condition		
Nutrition Oral		
Parenteral		
Output		

Assessment	Findings	Normal or Abnormal? (list significances if abnormal)
Behavior		
Signs of distress		
Needs		
Support		
Understanding		
Activity		

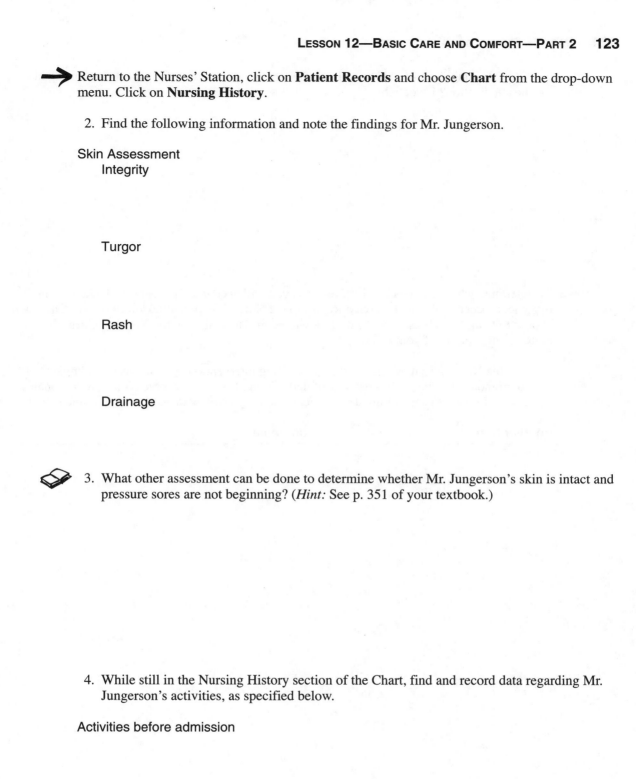

→ Return to the Nurses' Station, click on **Patient Records** and choose **Chart** from the drop-down menu. Click on **Nursing History**.

2. Find the following information and note the findings for Mr. Jungerson.

Skin Assessment
    Integrity

    Turgor

    Rash

    Drainage

3. What other assessment can be done to determine whether Mr. Jungerson's skin is intact and pressure sores are not beginning? (*Hint:* See p. 351 of your textbook.)

4. While still in the Nursing History section of the Chart, find and record data regarding Mr. Jungerson's activities, as specified below.

Activities before admission

Activity ordered during hospitalization

Level of personal care before admission

5. Will Mr. Jungerson be able to maintain his preadmission level of personal care during his hospitalization? If not, why?

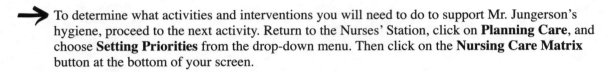 To determine what activities and interventions you will need to do to support Mr. Jungerson's hygiene, proceed to the next activity. Return to the Nurses' Station, click on **Planning Care**, and choose **Setting Priorities** from the drop-down menu. Then click on the **Nursing Care Matrix** button at the bottom of your screen.

6. Use the Nursing Care Matrix to find the nursing interventions you will need to implement to promote Mr. Jungerson's activity of daily living. List these interventions with rationales below. Be sure to keep in mind the patient's activity level, pain level, and emotional status.

Intervention   **Rationale**

7. Review Chapter 17 of your textbook for more interventions that you will need to implement to support Mr. Jungerson's hygiene and comfort. List them below.

8. What type of hygiene care will be necessary for you to implement? List specific care for each area below.

Bathing

Skin care

Hair care

Shaving

Nails and feet care

Bedmaking

9. What part(s) of these activities can Mr. Jungerson do himself? Why do you think he can do these?

Bathing

Skin care

Hair care

Shaving

Nails and feet care

Bedmaking

10. What parts of Mr. Jungerson's skin may be more susceptible to possible pressure sores or skin breakdown? Why?

11. What can you do to prevent pressure sore formation and skin breakdown from occurring?

12. What reinforcement of patient teaching regarding required adaptation in the performance of activities of daily living will you need to do for Mr. Jungerson?

LESSON 13

Basic Care and Comfort— Part 3

Client Need Categories: Palliative Care, Nonpharmacological Pain Interventions, and Rest and Sleep

Reading Assignment: Cultural and Ethnic Considerations (Chapter 7)
Pain Control, Comfort, Rest, and Sleep (Chapter 15)
Mathematics Review and Medication Administration (Chapter 22)

Patient: James Story, Room 512

Objectives

1. Apply heat and cold treatment as appropriate for your patient.
2. Assist with planning care for your patient with anticipated or actual alterations in comfort.
3. Check your patient's discomfort and pain level.
4. Check your patient's response to interventions that promote comfort.
5. Incorporate aspects of complementary and alternative medicine into patient care according to practice setting guidelines.
6. Monitor your patient for nonverbal signs of pain and discomfort.
7. Provide nonpharmacologic interventions for pain relief.
8. Recognize cultural differences in perception of and response to pain.

Introduction

Pain is a dreaded and unpleasant sensory and emotional experience for your patients. It is important to remember that pain is very subjective. The patient's description of pain needs to be accepted and dealt with accordingly. Patients will have different reactions to their pain, and treatment must be very individualized. The objective of pain management is to keep the patient comfortable consistently. Your role as a nurse is to establish a trusting relationship and provide assurance to your patient that you will assist him or her in a variety of methods to deal with the pain. This lesson will direct you through exercises of pain assessment and treatment to promote rest and sleep.

CD-ROM Activity

Insert *Virtual Clinical Excursions—General Hospital* Disk 2 in your CD-ROM drive and click on the **Shortcut to VCE** icon on your computer's desktop. Enter the hospital by clicking on the front doors. Once inside the lobby, click on the elevator and go to the Intensive Care Unit (Floor 5). When you arrive at the floor, click on the **Nurses' Station**; then double-click on the **Supervisor's (Login) Computer**. Sign in to work with James Story in Room 512 for the 07:00–08:29 period of care. Listen to the Case Overview and read your Assignment before returning to the Nurses' Station. In the upper left corner of the Nurses' Station screen, click on **Patient Care** and choose **Data**

Collection from the drop-down menu. Click on the various buttons and parts of the body model on the left and observe the nurse carrying out the physical assessment of James Story.

1. Briefly review the Data Collection to become familiar with James Story. Check the patient's discomfort, pain level, and nonverbal signs of pain. Make notes below as needed.

Notes

2. Record your findings for the following areas from the physical assessment.

Initial Observations

Vital Signs
    Blood pressure

    Heart rate

    Respiratory rate

    Pain assessment (rating and characteristics)

Upper Extremities
    Neurologic

IV

Wound Condition

Behavior Signs

Physiologic Signs

Ability to Sleep

3. Complete an example Chart entry that shows the results of your assessment. Be sure to use correct documentation principles.

→ Return to the Nurses' Station, click on **Planning Care** and choose **Problem Identification** from the drop-down menu. Read the Preceptor Note to answer the first part of question 3. Then return to the Nurses' Station, click again on **Planning Care**, and select **Setting Priorities**. Click on **Nursing Care Matrix** and use this resource to complete question 4.

4. Review the nursing diagnoses listed in the Preceptor Note and pick the ones that pertain to Mr. Story's pain and comfort level. List these below. Now determine what interventions you can implement for him. (*Hint:* If you need help, refer to Chapter 15 of your textbook for appropriate interventions.)

Nursing Diagnosis   **Interventions**

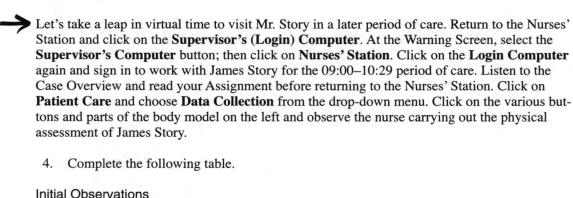 Let's take a leap in virtual time to visit Mr. Story in a later period of care. Return to the Nurses' Station and click on the **Supervisor's (Login) Computer**. At the Warning Screen, select the **Supervisor's Computer** button; then click on **Nurses' Station**. Click on the **Login Computer** again and sign in to work with James Story for the 09:00–10:29 period of care. Listen to the Case Overview and read your Assignment before returning to the Nurses' Station. Click on **Patient Care** and choose **Data Collection** from the drop-down menu. Click on the various buttons and parts of the body model on the left and observe the nurse carrying out the physical assessment of James Story.

4. Complete the following table.

Initial Observations

Vital Signs
    Blood pressure

    Heart rate

    Respiratory rate

    Pain assessment (rating and characteristics)

Upper Extremities
    Neurologic

IV

Wound Condition

Behavior Signs

Physiologic Signs

Ability to Sleep

→ Return to the Nurses' Station, click on **Patient Records**, and choose **EPR** from the drop-down menu. Enter the password—**nurse2b**—and click on **Access Records**. Record your findings from the physical assessment of Mr. Story. Remember to click on the checkmark in the lower right side of the screen when entering data. Refer to the **Getting Started** section in the front of this workbook for specific instructions on how to chart findings in the EPR.

6. What will be your next action to improve Mr. Story's comfort level? What nonpharmacologic interventions for pain relief can you use to make him more comfortable? (*Hint:* Refer to Chapter 15 in your textbook for suggestions).

7. What aspects of complementary and alternative medicine can you incorporate into Mr. Story's care according to practice setting guidelines?

➤ Return to the Nurses' Station, click on **Patient Records**, and select **MAR**.

8. What medications are ordered for Mr. Story's pain? List them below. Next to each, list the purpose, onset, duration, and side effects. (*Note:* Answers will vary according to what you decide is important to remember.)

Drug	Purpose	Onset	Duration	Side Effects

9. What nursing interventions can you implement in regard to management of Mr. Story's pain level with these medications?

Morphine

Acetaminophen

10. Choose what you think are the five most likely cultural or ethnic groups that you will encounter in taking care of patients where you will be practicing. Make a chart below that will assist you in the future in caring for patients with cultural differences in perception of and response to pain. (*Hint:* Refer to Chapter 7 of your textbook for assistance.)

Cultural or Ethnic Group   **Pain Perception and Responses**

Basic Care and Comfort— Part 4

Client Need Categories: Mobility/Immobility

Reading Assignment: Safety (Chapter 13)

Body Mechanics and Patient Mobility (Chapter 14)

Patient: Paul Jungerson, Room 602

Objectives

1. After considering your patient's mobility level, assist in teaching the patient to change position frequently.
2. Identify your patient's complication(s) of immobility.
3. Take action to maintain your patient's skin integrity.
4. Lift, transfer, transport, position, and assist your patient with ambulation using correct body mechanisms.
5. Monitor your patient's responses to:
   a. Immobility.
   b. Interventions for prevention of complication.
6. Monitor your patient's mobility, gait, and strength.
7. Provide assistance with prescribed exercises.

Introduction

When active patients are hospitalized, they often experience the effects of immobility, the alteration of a person's ability to more around freely. Immobility affects many systems of the human body and thus predisposes patients to the development of many complications. Interventions to prevent complications of immobility must be based on each patient's medical condition and abilities. The nurse's role is to promote physical health and well-being of the patient as health alterations occur. This lesson will direct you through activities that build you skills in mobility assessment, maintenance of wellness, and prevention of immobility by implementing movement needs for the patient.

CD-ROM Activity

Insert *Virtual Clinical Excursions—General Hospital* Disk 2 in your CD-ROM drive and click on the **Shortcut to VCE** icon on your computer's desktop. Enter the hospital by clicking on the front doors. Once inside the lobby, click on the elevator and go to the Medical-Surgical/Telemetry Floor (Floor 6). When you arrive at the floor, click on the **Nurses' Station**; then double-click on the **Supervisor's (Login) Computer**. Sign in to work with Paul Jungerson Room 602 for the 09:00–10:29 period of care. Listen to the Case Overview and read your Assignment before returning to the Nurses' Station. In the upper left corner of the Nurses' Station screen, click on

Patient Care and choose **Data Collection** from the drop-down menu. Click on the various buttons and parts of the body model on the left and observe the nurse carrying out the physical assessment of Paul Jungerson.

1. Complete the form below. The purpose of this form is to retain important information to refer to during your care. Be as specific as you need, but don't record everything, since it is already in the patient's Chart.

Patient's Name	Age	Diagnosis
Medical History	Surgery	Current Medications Last pain med
Assessment Information	IV	Wound/Dressing
Activity and Positioning	Other Pertinent Information	

One of the first actions you need to do is determine what activities Mr. Jungerson is able to tolerate. These activities will depend on the physician's orders, as well as the patient's diagnosis and state of wellness. The patient's current mobility, gait, and strength must be assessed, as well as his mobility before admission, current abilities, and what the physician has ordered.

→ Return to the Nurses' Station, click on **Patient Records**, and choose **Chart** from the drop-down menu. Click on **Nursing History** and answer the following questions.

2. What happened to Mr. Jungerson that is causing him to have discomfort in his left ankle?

3. Indicate whether or not Mr. Jungerson is able to perform the following daily activities of living independently.

Eating

Dressing

Ambulating

Toileting

Bathing

Grooming

4. What limits does Mr. Jungerson have on his mobility?

5. What assistive devices does Mr. Jungerson use?

6. What type of muscular weakness or fatigue does Mr. Jungerson have?

7. Does he have any swelling, redness, or warmth around joints or over muscles?

8. What type of gait does Mr. Jungerson have?

9. Are there any changes in the range of motion in his limbs?

10. From your answers to the previous questions, what can you determine about Mr. Jungerson's mobility before admission?

11. Mr. Jungerson has been in the hospital since last Friday around 11:00 a.m. What has his activity been during each day of his hospitalization? Be specific.

Friday

Saturday

Sunday

Monday

Tuesday

12. From your answer to question 11, what can you determine about Mr. Jungerson's mobility since admission?

Return to the Nurses' Station, click on **Planning Care**, and choose **Setting Priorities** from the drop-down menu. Click on **Nursing Care Matrix** at the bottom of your screen.

13. Consider Mr. Jungerson's response to his immobility and identify whether or not he is at risk to develop each of the complications listed below and on the next page. Using the Nursing Care Matrix, identify interventions that could prevent each complication. (*Hint:* If you need additional help, refer to Chapter 14 in your textbook.)

Complications	Mr. Jungerson at Risk for Development?	Interventions to Prevent Complication
Muscle and bone atrophy		
Contractures		
Decubitus ulcers/ pressure sores		
Constipation		
Urinary tract infection/ retention		
Disuse osteoporosis (easily fractured)		
Hypostatic pnuemonia		
Deep vein thrombosis		

Complications	Mr. Jungerson at Risk for Development?	Interventions to Prevent Complication
Pulmonary embolism		
Anorexia		
Insomnia		
Asthenia		
Disorientation		

14. Explain why each activity below and on the next page will help Mr. Jungerson to prevent complications from immobility. Be sure to include what specific activities will prevent complications. Make a short list of steps that will assist you when you offer care to him during your assigned time.

Positioning and movement of Mr. Jungerson while he is in bed

Transferring to a chair

Range of motion

15. You will assist in teaching Mr. Jungerson about the need to change position frequently to avoid the following complications. For each complication listed below and on the next page, identify appropriate patient teaching interventions, keeping in mind his mobility level. (*Hint:* Refer to Chapter 14 of your textbook for assistance.)

Complication	Patient Teaching Interventions to Prevent Complication
Muscle and bone atrophy	

Contractures

Complication	Patient Teaching Interventions to Prevent Complication
Decubitus ulcers/ pressure sores	
Constipation	
Urinary tract infection/ retention	
Disuse osteoporosis (easily fractured)	
Hypostatic pnuemonia	
Deep vein thrombosis	
Pulmonary embolism	
Anorexia	
Insomnia	
Asthenia	
Disorientation	

LESSON **15**

Basic Care and Comfort—
Part 5

Client Need Categories: Assistive Devices
Reading Assignment: Safety (Chapter 13)
　　　　　　　　　　　Body Mechanics and Patient Mobility (Chapter 14)

Patient: Elizabeth Washington, Room 604

Objectives

1. Assist your patient with assistive devices for ambulation.
2. Contribute to appropriate management of your patient using assistive devices.
3. Review correct use of assistive devices with your patient and family.
4. Assess your patient for communication problems.
5. Provide alternative methods for communication for your patient as appropriate

Introduction

When active patients are hospitalized, they are often at risk for complications related to immobility. Immobility, the alteration of a person's ability to more around freely, affects many systems of the human body and predisposes the patient to the development of many complications. Interventions to prevent complications of immobility must be based on each patient's medical condition and abilities. Often the patient requires the use of assistive devices for ambulation. The nurse's role is to promote mobility for the patient who uses assistive devices. Frequently, these devices are also needed after the patient leaves the hospital. Teaching the patient and family about the use of assistive devices is an important intervention. This lesson will direct you through activities that will build you skills in assessing a patient using assistive devices and teaching the patient and family about the importance of mobility and the use of assistive devices.

CD-ROM Activity

Insert *Virtual Clinical Excursions—General Hospital* Disk 2 in your CD-ROM drive and click on the **Shortcut to VCE** icon on your computer's desktop. Enter the hospital by clicking on the front doors. Once inside the lobby, click on the elevator and go to the Medical-Surgical/Telemetry Floor (Floor 6). When you arrive at the floor, click on the **Nurses' Station**; then double-click on the **Supervisor's (Login) Computer**. Sign in to work with Elizabeth Washington in Room 604 for the 11:00–12:29 period of care. Listen to the Case Overview and read your Assignment before returning to the Nurses' Station. In the upper left corner of the Nurses' Station screen, click on **Patient Care** and choose **Data Collection** from the drop-down menu. Click on the various buttons and parts of the body model on the left and observe the nurse carrying out the physical assessment of Ms. Washington.

147

1. Complete the following short form based on the physical assessment of Elizabeth Washington. This form should meet your needs for retaining information to use during your care. Be as specific as you need, but don't write everything, since it is already in the patient's Chart.

Patient's Name	Age	Diagnosis
Medical History	Surgery	Current Medications
Assessment Information	IV	Wound/Dressing
Activity and Positioning	Other Pertinent Information	

→ Return to the Nurses' Station, click on **Patient Records**, and choose **Chart** from the drop-down menu. Review the information in Ms. Washington's Nursing History, Physician Orders, and Progress Notes regarding her activity level.

2. Provide data for the following areas to determine Ms. Washington's mobility level.

Range of motion

Muscle strength

Gait

Posture

Current activity order

3. While still in Ms. Washington's Chart, click on the Social Services tab. Record notes below about what mobility needs have been determined for Ms. Washington.

4. Referring to Chapter 13 of your textbook, identify the assistive devices that Ms. Washington will need for ambulation. List safety interventions necessary for each device.

Assistive Device	Safety Interventions

5. With the information that you have gathered thus far, review the patient teaching that social services has given Ms. Washington and her family. Below, make a short list of topics that you will need to ask her and her family about each assistive device. For each teaching point, identify what response from the patient and/or family would indicate that they understand how to use the device safely.

Patient Teaching Point	Response from Patient and/or Family That Would Indicate Understanding

6. Ms. Washington has asked you to help her to the bathroom. Describe how you would help her and what type of assistive device should be in the bathroom. Why?

7. What behaviors indicate that Ms. Washington has not been able to incorporate the new information into her daily mobility activities?

8. You have had to repeat the same sentence three times now because Ms. Washington continues to ask you to repeat it. How can you help her understand what you are saying?

Pharmacologic Therapies—Part 1

Client Need Categories: Medication Administration and Pharmacological Actions)
Reading Assignment: Mathematics Review and Medication Administration
(Chapter 22)

Patients: James Story, Room 512
Elizabeth Washington, Room 604

Objectives

1. Administer medications correctly.
2. Determine your patient's need for administration of PRN medications.
3. Document medication administration.
4. Identify medication administration schedule.
5. Maintain controlled substances according to legal statutes.
6. Monitor your patient's use of medications.
7. Monitor the effects of medications.
8. Obtain information on prescribed medications from reference materials.
9. Review your patient's Chart for changes in medication regime.
10. Use the "six rights" when administering medications.

Introduction

The nurse must implement care related to medications that are ordered by the physician. To do this safely, you must be able to calculate the correct dosage and know the uses, pharmacologic actions, expected effects, side effects, and adverse reactions of each medication that is administered. Every patient will react differently to medication, and the nurse must be watchful of possible complications secondary to drug administration. This lesson will direct you through the techniques for administering prescribed medication safely.

CD-ROM Activity

Insert *Virtual Clinical Excursions—General Hospital* Disk 2 in your CD-ROM drive and click on the **Shortcut to VCE** icon on your computer's desktop. Enter the hospital by clicking on the front doors. Once inside the lobby, click on the elevator and go to the Intensive Care Unit (Floor 5). When you arrive at the floor, click on the **Nurses' Station**; then double-click on the **Supervisor's (Login) Computer**. Sign in to work with James Story in Room 602 for the 09:00–10:29 period of care. Listen to the Case Overview and read your Assignment before returning to the Nurses' Station. In the upper left corner of the Nurses' Station screen, click on **Patient Care** and choose **Data Collection** from the drop-down menu. Click on the various buttons and parts of the body model on the left and observe the nurse carrying out the physical assessment of James Story.

153

1. Complete the following short form to retain important information to use during your care of Mr. Story. Be as specific as you need, but don't try to write everything.

Patient's Name	Age	Diagnosis
Medical History	Surgery	Current Medications
		Last pain med
Assessment Information	IV	Wound/Dressing
Activity and Positioning	Other Pertinent Information	

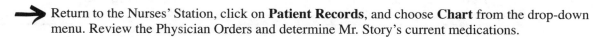

In order to correctly and safely administer medications, you need to know what has been ordered for Mr. Story and any possible contraindications for administration of those drugs. You also need to identify the medication administration schedule for this patient.

→ Return to the Nurses' Station, click on **Patient Records**, and choose **Chart** from the drop-down menu. Review the Physician Orders and determine Mr. Story's current medications.

 2. Complete the table below by first listing the drugs ordered for Mr. Story. For each drug, be sure to include the route, dosage, frequency, and any special directions. In the second column, identify why Mr. Story is receiving each medication. (*Hint:* Refer to Chapter 22 of your textbook and your drug reference book. This information may also be listed on the MAR.)

Drug, Route, Dosage, Frequency, Special Directions (including any data collection needed before drug administration)	Why Mr. Story Is Receiving This Medication

3. For each drug you listed in question 2, identify what action you expect and why that action occurs. (*Hint:* Refer to a drug handbook for help.)

Drug, Route, Dosage, Frequency, Special Directions	Action of Each Drug and Why That Action Occurs

4. Now list the nursing interventions needed for each of the drugs ordered for Mr. Story. (*Hint:* Refer to a drug handbook for specific interventions.)

Drug, Route, Dosage, Frequency, Special Directions	Nursing Interventions

Mr. Story is receiving medication to control his blood sugar, which is elevated. You will need to consult the Physician Orders for monitoring Mr. Story's blood glucose level and then find the order for the sliding scale coverage of insulin.

→ Return to the Physician Orders in Mr. Story's Chart.

  5. Complete the following orders.

Physician Orders for monitoring Mr. Story's blood glucose

Date ordered

Was order put on Kardex?   MAR?

Frequency of monitoring

Does this monitoring continue after the surgical procedure?

Where can you find this information?

  6. What is the policy in your clinical facility for renewing orders after surgery and procedures?

  7. Once you are certain that the order is correct or you have received a correct order, how much insulin would you give for each of the blood glucose levels below, according to the Physician Order given for Mr. Story on Monday at 07:00.

Sample Sliding Scale Coverage

Time	Blood Glucose Level	Sliding Scale Regular Insulin Coverage	Other Nursing Interventions Needed
0600	368		
0800	180		
1000	425		
1200	251		
1400	250		
1600	325		

8. On the sample MAR below, chart any medication(s) you would give during your assigned time of care (09:00–10:29) for Mr. Story using the sample sliding scale coverage table you completed for question 7. (*Hint:* Refer to Mr. Story's MAR for these orders, keeping in mind his pain level, routine medications, PRN medications, and sliding scale. Be sure to include any data collection needed before giving the medications.)

Patient: James Story	MRN: 123456	Room: 211	Date: Tuesday
Medication Administration Record			
Medication	2300–0700	0700–1500	1500–2300

Time	Stat/PRN	Injection Code

Nurses	Signature 2300-0700	Initials	Signature 0700-1500	Initials
Nurses	Signature 1500-2300	Initials	Signature	Initials

9. Were there any ordered medications that you could not give? If so, which? Why could you not give the medication(s)? What action do you need to take to ensure that Mr. Story receives what he needs?

10. Document other nursing interventions that are needed to regulate Mr. Story's blood glucose. (*Hint:* Refer to a drug handbook for other nursing interventions for hyperglycemia management.)

11. Refer to Chapter 22 of your textbook and list the six rights that you would follow if you were to give any medications to Mr. Story.

(1)

(2)

(3)

(4)

(5)

(6)

12. Mr. Story has an order for morphine sulfate 2 mg IV q2h PRN pain. Describe how you would maintain this controlled substance according to legal statutes and local facility policies. If unfamiliar with this process, list where you might find the correct procedure.

13. List the correct steps for counting or ensuring that all controlled substances were given to the patients and that none are missing at the end of your shift.

You are now ready to work with a new patient. You will need to go to a different floor to visit this patient. Return to the Nurses' Station and click on the **Login Computer**. Then select the **Supervisor's Computer** button, followed by the **Nurses' Station** button. You are now logged out. Click on the elevator and go to the Medical-Surgical/Telemetry Floor (Floor 6). Click on the **Supervisor's (Login) Computer** and sign in to work with Elizabeth Washington in Room 604 for the 09:00–10:29 period of care. Listen to the Case Overview and read your Assignment before returning to the Nurses' Station. Review Ms. Washington's MAR as needed to complete question 14.

 14. You will be giving Ms. Washington all of her medications that are due during this period of care, except those given by IV. There are multidose bottles of medications in Ms. Washington's medication drawer (as listed below and on the next page). Calculate the current doses for each of Ms. Washington's medication orders and ensure that all drugs are given as ordered for your assigned time. For each drug listed, indicate the dosage you would give. Your answers will depend on what type of dosage calculation you use. (*Hint:* See Chapter 22 of your textbook for assistance as needed.)

Medication Available	Medication Order and Calculation	Correct Dosage/Pills
Hydrochlorothiazide 50-mg tablets (bottle of 10 pills)		
Docusate sodium 50 mg in unit-dose packages		
Enoxaparin 120 mg/1 ml vial		
Multivitamin and Fe 300 mg/tablet in unit-dose packages		

Medication Available	Medication Order and Calculation	Correct Dosage/Pills
Montelukast sodium 10 mg/tablet (bottle of 10 pills)		
Certirizine 10 mg/tablet (bottle of 10 pills)		

15. What actions do you need to take to ensure that all Ms. Washington's ordered medications are available and are given correctly?

16. Chart the medications that you have given Ms. Washington.

Patient: Washington, Eliz MRN: 4873017 Room: 604 Date: Tuesday			
Medication Administration Record			
Medication	2300–0700	0700–1500	1500–2300

Time	Stat/PRN	Injection Code	

Nurses	Signature 2300-0700	Initials	Signature 0700-1500	Initials
Nurses	Signature 1500-2300	Initials	Signature	Initials

Pharmacologic Therapies—Part 2

Client Need Categories: Adverse Effects, Expected Effects, and Side Effects
Reading Assignment: Mathematics Review and Medication Administration (Chapter 22)

Patients: Julia Parker, Room 608

Objectives

1. Review and use resources for medication administration, outlining purposes, doses, side effects, and other considerations.
2. Identify actual and potential incompatibilities of medications prescribed to your patient.
3. Monitor your patient's response for actual or potential side effects of medications.
4. Withhold medications if your patient is experiencing adverse reactions.
5. Document side effects and/or adverse effects of medications administered to your patient.
6. Implement procedures to counteract adverse effects of medications.

Introduction

The nurse must implement care related to medications that are ordered by the physician. In order to do this safely, you must follow the six rights during administration. The nurse must also be aware of uses, pharmacologic actions, expected effects, side effects, and adverse reactions of each medication administered. Patients will react differently to medication, and the nurse must be watchful of possible complications secondary to drug administration. Implementation of procedures to counteract adverse effects or potential complications due to the drug's effect on the patient need to be initiated as soon as possible. This lesson will direct you through activities that assist you to recognize adverse reactions and identify interventions to implement in response to these undesirable effects.

CD-ROM Activity

Insert *Virtual Clinical Excursions—General Hospital* Disk 2 in your CD-ROM drive and click on the **Shortcut to VCE** icon on your computer's desktop. Enter the hospital by clicking on the front doors. Once inside the lobby, click on the elevator and go to the Medical-Surgical/Telemetry Floor (Floor 6). When you arrive at the floor, click on the **Nurses' Station**; then double-click on the **Supervisor's (Login) Computer**. Sign in to work with Julia Parker in Room 608 for the 09:00–10:29 period of care. Listen to the Case Overview and read your Assignment before returning to the Nurses' Station. In the upper left corner of the Nurses' Station screen, click on **Patient Care** and choose **Data Collection** from the drop-down menu. Click on the various buttons and parts of the body model on the left and observe the nurse carrying out the physical assessment of Julia Parker.

1. Complete the short form below. This form should meet your needs for retaining information to use during your care. Be as specific as you need, but don't try to write everything.

Patient's Name	Age	Diagnosis
Medical History	Surgery	Current Medications Last pain med
Assessment Information VS (include pain rating and O_2 sat)	IV	Wound/Dressing
Activity and Positioning	Other Pertinent Information	

In order to correctly and safely administer medications, you need to know what has been ordered for Ms. Parker and any possible contraindications for administration of those drugs. You also need to identify the medication administration schedule for her.

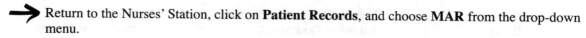 Return to the Nurses' Station, click on **Patient Records**, and choose **MAR** from the drop-down menu.

 2. Complete the table below by listing Ms. Parker's current medications. Be sure to include route, dosage, frequency, and any special directions. In the second column, identify why she is receiving each medication. (*Hint:* Refer to Chapter 22 of your textbook and your drug reference book for assistance.)

Drug, Route, Dosage, Frequency, Special Directions (including recommended data collection)	Why Ms. Parker Is Receiving This Medication

3. For each medication that Ms. Parker is receiving, list the side effects and possible adverse reactions. Identify actual and potential incompatibilities of the medications prescribed for her. (*Hint:* Refer to Chapter 22 of your textbook and your drug reference book for help.)

Drug	Side Effects and Possible Adverse Reactions	Incompatibilities

4. Which two drugs from the list above might be given together? Why?

➡ Return to the Nurses' Station, click on **Patient Care**, and choose **Data Collection** from the drop-down menu. Click on the various buttons and parts of the body model on the left and observe the nurse carrying out the physical assessment of Julia Parker.

5. Take notes about Ms. Parker's condition on the following assessments based on the findings from the 09:00 Data Collection. Indicate the significance of each finding.

Assessment	09:00 Findings	Significance
Vital Signs		
Blood pressure		
SpO$_2$		
Heart rate		
Respiratory rate		
Temperature		
Pain assessment		
Behavior		
Signs of distress		
Needs		
Support		
Understanding		
Activity		

6. Describe Ms. Parker's condition at this time.

7. Is your answer to question 6 related to any of the medications that Ms. Parker currently is taking? Why or why not?

8. What actions should you take?

18

Pharmacologic Therapies—Part 3

Client Need Categories: Complicating Adverse Effects and Side Effects

Reading Assignment: Mathematics Review and Medication Administration (Chapter 22)

Patients: Julia Parker, Room 608

Objectives

1. Identify actual and potential incompatibilities of medications prescribed to your patient.
2. Document your patient's responses to action taken to counteract adverse effects of medications.
3. Monitor your patient's response for actual or potential side effects of medications.
4. Withhold medications if your patient is experiencing adverse reactions.
5. Document side effects and/or adverse effects of medications administered to your patient.
6. Implement procedures to counteract adverse effects of medications.
7. Notify primary health care provider about actual/potential incompatibilities and side/adverse effects of your patient's medications.
8. Review patient teaching on management of side effects of self-administered medications.

Introduction

The nurse must implement care related to medications ordered by the physician. In order to do this safely, you must follow the six rights of medication administration. You must also be aware of uses, pharmacologic actions, expected effects, side effects, and adverse reactions of each medication that is administered. Patients react differently to medication, and the nurse must be watchful of possible complications secondary to drug administration. Implementation of procedures to counteract adverse effects or potential complications due to the drug's effect on the patient need to be initiated as soon as possible. This lesson will direct you through activities designed to assist you in recognizing adverse reactions and identifying interventions to implement in response to these undesirable effects.

CD-ROM Activity

Insert *Virtual Clinical Excursions—General Hospital* Disk 2 in your CD-ROM drive and click on the **Shortcut to VCE** icon on your computer's desktop. Enter the hospital by clicking on the front doors. Once inside the lobby, click on the elevator and go to the Medical-Surgical/Telemetry Floor (Floor 6). When you arrive at the floor, click on the **Nurses' Station**; then double-click on the **Supervisor's (Login) Computer**. Sign in to work with Julia Parker in Room 608 for the 09:00–10:29 period of care. Listen to the Case Overview and read your Assignment before

171

returning to the Nurses' Station. In the upper left corner of the Nurses' Station screen, click on **Patient Care** and choose **Data Collection** from the drop-down menu. Click on the various buttons and parts of the body model on the left and observe the nurse carrying out the physical assessment of Julia Parker.

1. Complete the short form below. This form should meet your needs for retaining information to use during your care. Be as specific as you need, but don't write everything.

Patient's Name	Age	Diagnosis
Medical History	Surgery	Current Medications Last pain med
Assessment Information VS (include pain rating and O_2 sat)	IV	Wound/Dressing
Activity and Positioning	Other Pertinent Information	

In order to correctly and safely administer medications, you need to know what has been ordered for Ms. Parker and any possible contraindications for administration of those drugs. You will also need to identify a medication administration schedule for her.

 Return to the Nurses' Station, click on **Patient Records**, and choose **MAR** from the drop-down menu.

 2. Complete the table below by listing Ms. Parker's current medication orders. For each drug, be sure to include route, dosage, frequency, and any special directions. In the second column, identify why she is receiving each medication. (*Hint:* Refer to Chapter 22 of your textbook and your drug reference book. If you have done this exercise during another lesson, find it and keep it handy for the rest of this lesson.)

Drug, Route, Dosage, Frequency, Special Directions (including recommended data collection)	Why Ms. Parker Is Receiving This Medication

3. For each of the medications that Ms. Parker is receiving, list the side effects and possible adverse reactions. Also identify any incompatabilities (actual or potential) of the drugs ordered for her. (*Hint:* Refer to Chapter 22 of your textbook and your drug reference book. If you have done this during another lesson, review that exercise.)

Drug	Side Effects and Adverse Reactions	Incompatibilities

4. Which two drugs from the list in question 3 might be given together? Why?

→ Return to the Nurses' Station, click on **Patient Records**, and select **Chart**. Review Ms. Parker's Lab Reports and Progress Reports.

5. Based on your review of Ms. Parker's chart, determine whether she is having any expected side effects or adverse reactions from any of the medications ordered. (*Note:* This information may also be found in the EPR.) Identify the section of the Chart or EPR you used to make your determination.

6. What medications would you *not* give if the following symptoms were present? Why would you not give them?

Symptom	Medication(s) You Would Withhold	Why
Low blood glucose (80)		
Low blood pressure 90/50		
Diarrhea		
Bleeding of the gums		
Pulse rate 130		

7. If Ms. Parker were experiencing the following symptoms, what would you do in addition to withholding medication? Offer rationales for your actions.

Symptom	Other Action Needed, Including Rationale
Low blood sugar (80)	
Low blood pressure (90/50)	
Diarrhea	
Bleeding of the gums	
Pulse rate 130	

8. What patient teaching would you emphasis regarding these symptoms?

Symptom	Patient Teaching Emphasized
Low blood sugar (80)	
Low blood pressure (90/50)	
Diarrhea	
Bleeding of the gums	
Pulse rate 130	

9. On the sample MAR below, indicate how you would chart the medications that you with-held in question 7. (*Hint:* If needed, refer to the MAR as a guide. You may follow the policy used in any of your clinical facilities.)

Patient: Sample Patient	MRN: 123456	Room: 211	Date: Sample

Medication Administration Record

Medication	2300–0700	0700–1500	1500–2300

Time	Stat/PRN	Injection Code

Nurses	Signature 2300-0700	Initials	Signature 0700-1500	Initials
Nurses	Signature 1500-2300	Initials	Signature	Initials

Notes

Notes

Notes

Notes

Notes